The Status and Unchanging Names of The Corona Virus:
Why is it Still Here?

Dina S. Morris

ORIGIN

According to the majority of the world's most renowned experts on transmittable diseases, COVID-19, which is spreading across China, is likely to evolve into a widespread condition spreading across the globe. Its potential impact is truly terrifying. A pandemic, a widespread outbreak that extends across at least two continents, well cause global problems, including China and other countries, such as that of the United States,[1] which are in the process of imposing new restrictions on travel and quarantines.

Scientists cannot determine how fatal the new coronavirus is, and there's some concern about the extent of damage the virus could cause. There is, however, an increasing consensus that the pathogen is easily transmitted to people. It is believed that COVID-19 is more similar to the highly transmissible influenza than scientists' findings in its slower-moving viruses, SARS and MERS.

The number of confirmed cases of TB in the lab has grown over the last three weeks, from approximately 50 cases in China to nearly 17,000 across more than 23 nations. There were at least 360 fatalities. But specific epidemiological models forecast the total number of cases to be at least 100,000 or more. Although this growth isn't as rapid as that of measle, or fulfil a significant leap over what virologists saw when they saw

Researchers aren't yet able to pinpoint who is most at the risk f developing a serious or life-threatening illness and what triggers may help. Children are more likely than middle-aged or older men to contract serious illnesses. The majority of foreigners who have recently been to China are barred from entering the United States. Americans who have returned to Wuhan and the centre of the epidemic, Hubei Province, are held for two weeks. Health officials at the federal level advise Americans not to travel to China regardless.

This is a crucial public health issue that requires proactive action to safeguard the public has been taken and is being implemented by both the C.D.C. and the federal government. There are one or two cases within the U.S., and Americans' risk is low. We have learned about the virus and its spread so far.

CHAPTER 1

HUMAN CORONAVIRUS OUTBREAK 2020

As the year came to an end, reports surfaced from an unidentified outbreak of cause of pneumonia. The cases were located in Wuhan's Huanan Seafood Wholesale Market, China, selling live poultry, fish, and birds. The outbreak was first reported on 8th December, but it was only noticed at the end of December. The market was closed on 1 January 2020, and on 7 January, the coronavirus was identified by Chinese authorities. All suspected cases discovered were screened with active case finding and retrospective analysis. Around 300 cases reported in Wuhan were thought to be infected by this virus. Four of them died.

It is also believed that earlier similar illnesses, like SARS, result from live animal sales. Camels carry coronaviruses that cause MERS to human beings. The animal believed to be responsible for the latest coronavirus is unknown, and the collapse of the market for meat within Wuhan has made it difficult to research. Bats are a potential source because several viruses, including the coronavirus, have evolved to coexist. However, it is likely that an intermediate species passed the disease by bats and then humans.

Wuhan, a virology-focused centre in China, was well placed to identify and combat the outbreak. However, it has put China's preparedness for disease to the test in a region of the world that frequently recalls the 2003 severe coronavirus epidemic of an acute respiratory syndrome (SARS). The virus spread across China to 25 countries, infected over 8000 people, and killed approximately 800 before being kept at bay. In the current case, the speed with which the Chinese authorities announced the outbreak to the world community was commendable, proving that lessons learned from earlier outbreaks have been considered.

As the world's community reacts to the coronavirus outbreak caused by pneumonia in Wuhan, China, early and open data sharing-essential to its security is contingent on the confidence that the data is not used without proper attribution to the person made it.

How can you tell the Human Coronavirus, and What is it? How Dangerous is it?

Coronaviruses form a huge virus family that typically targets breathing organs. The name derives from the Latin word corona, which means crown. This is due to the spiky slit which surrounds the viruses. Like birds, bats, and cats, numerous species suffer from the illness. Seven species cause human illness, including SARS, Covid-19, and MERS.

SARS is believed to have originated from China, beginning with bats and then cats and eventually humans. MERS has been transmitted from camels to bats to Middle East humans. There is no way to determine where the Covid-19 originated from. As of now, animals in Wuhan, China, a town with a population of 11 million, are believed to have jumped in the last quarter of the year. However, researchers are still trying to discover their origins.

For the symptoms present, in between 10 and 30 % of cases, one of seven coronaviruses infect human beings, SARS and MERS, leading to severe pneumonia or even death. Other viruses, however, exhibit less serious effects, such as the common cold. Covid-19 can kill, but it's unknown what frequency or how it relates to the death rate in relation to SARS and MERS.

According to the Centre for Disease Control and Prevention, most patients suffer from cough, fever, and breathlessness symptoms. A preliminary analysis, released in The Lancet, offered even more details. The study examined only a small portion of the 41 patients from Wuhan who had confirmed Covid-19. The symptoms of fever, cough, exhaustion, and pain were the most frequent. However, vomiting, nausea vomiting, and coughing up mucus and blood were not as frequent. All were diagnosed with CT tests for pneumonia as well as lung problems. Thirteen people were rushed to an ICU concerning the serious illness, where six perished. On 22 January, most patients were released from the hospital (68 percent).

Recently, records are also being recorded of patients with mild symptoms, for instance, the people in the southern part of Germany. There's even evidence that these events are not symptomatic. Covid-19 may appear more similar to flu than SARS. Infections tend to be more serious when first discovered since people admitted to hospitals are often the sickest. But the latest virus appears less risky in comparison to the other two, SARS or MERS.

How Bad Could the Outbreak Be?

The novel coronavirus, like SARS, appears to be highly contagious. The severity of an outbreak depends on how fast and easy it is passed from one person to another. While the work is only beginning, researchers have calculated that every person who has the coronavirus may be infected by 1.5 to 3.5 people in other countries without effective containment measures. The virus could be almost as deadly as SARS, the corona-related virus circulating in China in 2003. It was stopped after 898 people were affected and 774 were killed. These respiratory viruses could travel through the air and be wrapped in tiny droplets created when a sick individual coughs, breathes, speaks, or coughs. A few droplets will fall within a few feet of the ground. This makes it more difficult for the disease to spread differently from viruses such as measles, tuberculosis, and chickenpox that can travel across the sky for hundred miles. However, it is more effective to detect than H.I.V. or hepatitis that is transmitted through direct contact with an affected person's bodily fluids.

If each person infected with the coronavirus can infect up to three others, it could be enough to perpetuate and grow the spread of the disease if nothing is implemented to decrease the spread. Compare that with the less harmful virus such as the seasonal flu. The flu-infected appear to spread the virus to 1.3 others. It may seem like a small difference, but the result is an astonishing contrast: there are only 45 people in the same scenario who might be affected.

The number of instances that are outside of China is very limited. However, reports have surfaced in several nations in the last few days, including in the United States, of citizens who haven't visited China. Furthermore, in 2003, amount of cases in China significantly exceeded the rate for SARS cases. The real amount of cases is certain to be much higher than what is officially verified through laboratory tests.

Many people are suspected of being infected at the Hubei province, where the outbreak began in the early 1990s, but they're not confirmed. Doctors report a shortage of testing equipment and medical. Residents find it extremely difficult to obtain the medical treatment they need to manage the coronavirus even detect them. Different epidemiological models predict that the number of cases will be around 100,00more. Experts have advised caution when making calculations for these numbers.

How Deadly is the Virus?

It's still difficult to determine. The fatality rate could be lower than 3 percent, and, despite that, it's much less than SARS. This is among the most important factors, and determining the fatality of an emerging virus is not easy. The fatal cases are often initially discovered, which could alter our understanding of how patients will be killed. A third of Wuhan's initial 41 patients were required to be admitted to an ICU, and many of them had symptoms of fever, severe cough, and shortness of breath. Pneumonia. An ophthalmologist cannot see patients with mild conditions. There are more deaths than we realize, and the mortality rate could be lower than originally believed.

However, there might be unreported deaths due to the virus. The Chinese cities at the centre of the epidemic are experiencing an acute shortage of tests kits and beds in hospitals, and many patients cannot see a doctor. There's some uncertainty regarding the presence of this virus and what it's doing. Initial indications suggest that the mortality rate for this particular virus is less than the other coronavirus MERS, which kills around 35 percent of affected individuals, and SARS, which kills approximately 10. All diseases connect to proteins on the lung cell's surface; however, MERS and SARS are more damaging to lung tissue.

In China's 17,000 patients, 82% suffered from moderate symptoms, 15% suffered from serious symptoms, and three percent were classified as critically ill. A mere 2 percent have been confirmed dead from illnesses. Most of those who passed away were older men who had chronic health problems. The virus can cause serious respiratory diseases (i.e., pneumonia) and death due to mild symptoms. Many deaths were among those older than 65 and treated for another chronic illness or disease. There is a chance that the fatality rate for each case is 2 percent (meaning two deaths from 100 cases confirmed), although it's still too early to provide any reliable information. If the number of undetected symptoms or cases with only mild symptoms turns out to be high, it could be less. If the virus becomes mutated, it can intensify. However, the death rate is usually lower than the rate of SARS (10 percent) and higher than that of seasonal influenza (less than 0.01 percentage).

Where Has the Virus Spread?

We aren't sure the exact mechanism by which Covid-19 is spread; however, we do have plenty of information on what happens when MERS, SARS, and other respiratory viruses can spread from person to person. It occurs most often due to the contact with droplets caused by coughing or sneezing. If a person is suffering from illness, coughs, or coughs, they release an odor, and when the droplets get into someone's eyes, nose, or even their mouths, they are infected. In some cases, a person can indirectly contract a respiratory infection "by touching droplets on surfaces and then touching mucosal membranes" within the eyes, mouth, and nose. Hand washing is a crucial aspect of health for the public, especially during an outbreak.

The virus spread quickly because it started in a hub for transportation. Wuhan is one of the most difficult places to have an outbreak. There are 11 million residents, more than the City of New York. On an average day, 3,500 passengers fly directly to cities in other countries from Wuhan. These cities have been among the first cities outside China to track virus cases. Wuhan is also a major transport hub within China connected via high-speed trains and local airlines that connect to Beijing, Shanghai, and other major cities. Up to 2 million people travelled by plane from Wuhan to other areas within China during November and October last year.

When the SARS outbreak of 2003, China was not as close as. Many workers are now moving across the country and internationally to Africa and other regions of Asia and Latin America, where China's Belt and Road Initiative is creating a massive infrastructure push. The movement of these workers poses a high chance of triggering outbreaks in countries with health care systems that are not equipped to deal with these outbreaks, like Zimbabwe, which is struggling with increasing poverty and economic turmoil.

Additionally, China has about four times as many travellers in the air and on trains as during the SARS outbreak. China made the bold move of imposing travel restrictions on the millions of people who live in Wuhan and the surrounding cities. However, experts warned that the lockout might be too late with limited access to medicines and food. Wuhan's mayor had confirmed that 5 million residents left the city before this year's Lunar New Year before the restrictions were put in place.

The Mode of Transmission

The Transmission Mode The mechanism by which Covid-19, a coronavirus, spreads is unknown. Current knowledge is based mostly on the knowledge gained from coronaviruses with similar characteristics. Coronaviruses comprise a huge group of viruses encountered in various animals, including cats, camels, goats, and bats. Rarely, animal coronavirus is transmitted to humans, and later they spread to people, including MERS, SARS, and recently, with Covid-19. Most respiratory infections are spread through coughing and sneezing. While the Chinese authorities initially dismissed the possibility of human-to-human transmission, the widespread and long-lasting transmission between individuals has been discovered. Chinese researchers have warned that infected people may transfer the disease to other people even before they get sick or develop any symptoms. Still, a research study showing asymptomatic transmission in Germany was criticized for being in error.

If people carry the virus with no symptoms or mild symptoms related to respiratory diseases, like back pain or headaches, this is a huge problem. People are out and about, heading to work or the church or gym, as well as breathing on or touching others who don't even know they're sick. Most of the time, the spread from person to person occurs in close contact (about 6 inches). It is believed that spreading between people occurs mostly through the respiratory droplets produced by an infected individual who coughs or sneezes. It's like how respiratory pathogens like influenza can apply. Droplets of this kind could land close to people's noses or mouths and then be breathed into the lung. It is unclear if a person can contract Covid-19 from touching a surface or an object with the virus and then touching their mouth or nose, or perhaps eyes is at present unclear. In general, people are believed to be the most susceptible to most respiratory viruses when they're symptoms-prone (the sickest).

It is crucial to remember that the speed of a virus spread can differ from one person to the next. Many viruses (such as measles) are extremely contagious; however other viruses aren't. There's much more to learn about the transmissibility, frequency, and aspects of Covid-19 and ongoing research. This data will assist in the risk assessment process further.

What Symptoms Should I Look Out For?

Signs of the infection include symptoms of this infection, including a heavy cough, fever, breathing problems, and shortness of breath. The condition causes lung lesions and pneumonia. The mild cases can resemble the flu or a cold, making it difficult to recognize. Patients might have other signs, like digestive issues or diarrhea. It is well-known that the period of incubation, the time between the first exposure to the onset manifestations—can be in the range of 10 days to two weeks.

Consult your doctor If you are suffering from an illness such as a cough or fever and recently travelled to China or stayed with someone who has. Contact them first to prepare for your visit and take measures to ensure that you are not exposed to other patients or staff.

How Time-consuming Does It Take to Reveal Symptoms?

The coronavirus that is being developed has symptoms between 2 and 14 days, which allows the illness to go unnoticed. It has been reported to affect individuals with no or minimal symptoms to those who are seriously ill and dying due to confirmed Covid-19 infections. Signs and symptoms can include:

- Fever
- Cough
- Breathing shortness

This is based on what was previously known as the MERS virus incubation. The time it takes for symptoms to manifest after the infection can be crucial in preventing and controlling. The duration is known as incubation, and this period assists health authorities in identifying people who may be exposed. However, if the incubation duration is too long or short, it might be difficult to follow these steps.

A variety of diseases, including influenza, can be treated with a short duration of two to three days of incubation. As long as they don't show flu symptoms, individuals can shed infectious viruses, making it difficult to distinguish and identify individuals with the virus. However, SARS had an incubation time of around five days. It took anywhere from four to five days after the symptoms began before the virus could be transferred to patients and allowed officials the time to end the infection and control the outbreak effectively.

The top executives at the Centres for Disease Regulator and Prevention state that incubation for the coronavirus currently infected are between 2 and 14 days. However, the possibility that a person could contract the virus before symptoms appear is not certain, nor is it clear if the severity of the disease affects the speed with which patients can spread it. This is a concern because it could mean that the detection of the illness will remain elusive.

CORONAVIRUS - SARS

The year 2003 was when SARS began to be recognized for the first time as a distinctive coronavirus type. The cause of the virus has never been evident, but the first human cases can be traced to Guangdong Province in 2002. The virus later became a pandemic that led to more than 8,000 flu-like cases in 26 countries, with around 800 deaths. In contrast to SARS, the new outbreak is caused by a coronavirus, a group of common viruses ranging from the common cold to serious illnesses, like respiratory syndrome prevalent in the Middle East (MERS).

There is a reason why COVID-19 triggered alarm across the globe, but the memories of a fatal virus are also popping to the forefront in Asia. There are two elements common to the coronavirus circulating in China and the SARS outbreak. Both are part of the coronavirus group and are likely transferred from animals to human beings through a wet market. Coronaviruses are zoonotic, which means they can transmit from animals to humans. Because wet markets place humans and dead and alive animals-pigs, dogs, chickens, rats, civets, and much more-in proximity creating an interspecies leap could be simple for viruses to take advantage of.

Live-animal markets that are not properly regulated and poorly regulated with the illegal trade of animals provide a unique possibility for viruses to spread to humans from the wildlife they feed on. Bats were the primary hosts of SARS and, possibly, this coronavirus outbreak, too. They transmitted the virus to other animals through their saliva or poop and unintentionally passed it on to humans. Birds and bats are both considered potential pandemic reservoir species.

Three other epidemics (apart from the one that is SARS) were linked to bats over the past 45 years. They were the primary source of Ebola in 1976. Since then, it has killed over 13,500 people across multiple outbreaks. Middle Eastern respiratory syndrome, also known as MERS, has been reported in 28 countries, and the Nipah virus with a death rate of 78 percent. To many, the current outbreak is eerily like 2003, when the severe acute respiratory disorder (SARS) took over the nation and infected over 8,000 individuals and the deaths 774.

While an identical virus can trigger SARS and the Wuhan coronavirus and SARS, they're not the same. The two viruses are, in fact lining each other up. More confirmed Wuhan corona-related cases have overtaken the 2003 SARS outbreak on mainland China and several countries removed their residents from the area within the SARS outbreak. As per Chinese officials, there are reported infections of the disease across mainland China with the deaths of 132. In the week ending Tuesday, confirmed cases increased by around 1500, more than 30 percent. These numbers don't comprise Hong Kong and Macau, with only a few reported cases. There were at most 91 cases of the disease outside the mainland of China.

However, there were 5 327 confirmed disease cases in mainland China in the 2003 SARS outbreak, which resulted in 349 deaths. Experts have previously believed that Wuhan virus figures could be under-reported, making the coronavirus, a novel virus, more invasive and less deadly than SARS.

Chinese authorities have confirmed a suspected instance of Wuhan disease in Tibet, the region that was once the only location to avoid spreading the virus. If it is approved, the spread of the virus to Tibet despite rigorous traveller security and the shut-down of tourist attractions will rekindle questions about the ease with which the virus could be transmitted, especially if individuals are not symptomatic.

Each of the cases of SARS and Wuhan originated in China, and both are believed to have come from markets for wild animals. In China, scientists have examined the Wuhan corona virus's genetic code with other coronaviruses and discovered it to be the closest to two bat coronaviruses. Experts have not confirmed the species of animal that caused the virus to spread to humans, but they have a few guesses. Researchers consider that coronaviruses that cause SARS were derived from a bat-based reservoir passed on to the civet cat. This wild animal is regarded as a treat in certain areas of southern China before spreading to humans.

This latest virus was identified as being related to the closed Huanan Seafood Wholesale Market located in Wuhan Wuhan, where various wildlife, such as snakes and raccoons, were available for purchase. Animals transmitted the coronavirus, possibly snakes, and later passed on to humans, perhaps bats. Further analysis of genetics discovered that the snakes looked like the genetic building blocks that comprise COVID-19. Researchers believe that a bat population could be contaminated with rats that transferred human beings with the disease when sold on the Wuhan Huanan Wholesale Seafood Market. In the wake of SARS, China has banned Civet cats from slaughter and consumption. China was going one step further with this one and announced that it would exclude all animal products sold to wild animals around the globe.

Yet, a second study that challenges the notion that the virus resulted from the Huanan Huanan wet market was published. According to Science and cited in an article published within The Lancet medical journal, Chinese scientists discovered that the first instance in COVID-19 in December did not connect to the market. In addition, 13 out of 41 cases they studied for coronavirus did not relate to the Huanan market. There is only one way for researchers to know where the virus came from is to collect DNA samples from animals sold in the market and bats, and snakes roamed in the region.

Number of Infections

More than 7,700 people have been affected by the first Wuhan coronavirus case reported in December. Contrast this with the fact that from November 2002 to July 2003, there were 898 confirmed cases of SARS. It took less than two months for people to become sick over nine months, about 75 percent of those patients diagnosed with SARS.

A lot has been confirmed; COVID-19 cases have already reached the amount of SARS infected between 2002 and 2003. Since the epidemic of China's SARS nearly 17 years ago, many things have changed. But some aspects haven't. Today, at least seven hundred and one cases are reported across mainland China compared to 5 327 cases confirmed of SARS on 16 August 2003, the Chinese Ministry of Health said the results.

Chinese domestic and international travel has been increasing rapidly since 2003, which could aid in spreading the disease faster. According to Chinese government figures, the number of tourists who travelled out of China increased by 16.6 million visits in 2003 and 149.7 million by 2018. It's important to note that this outbreak happened in China during the most difficult season- the Lunar New Year- where millions of people visit home to visit their family members. As of 27 January, it was reported that there had been 4,096 Wuhan tourists traveling abroad, according to Wuhan's Culture and Tourism office.

Number of Deaths

Seven hundred seventy-four people perished in the year 2003 SARS epidemic. In China, mainland China, and Hong Kong, most deaths occurred. At present, the virus has infected 170 people and, so far, most of them are in mainland China. When assessing the number of death rates, the most important factor to examine is the rate of death for cases, which measures the percentage of patients who die. The rate of fatality for COVID-19 stands at around 2 percent. This is substantially lower than the death rate of 9.6 percentage for SARS. It's also less than Middle East Respiratory Syndrome (MERS)—a different form of coronavirus with a 35% of cases fatality rate.

However, this estimate is only as reliable as the numbers reported. Many experts are concerned that they don't accurately estimate the number of people infected within China since tests kits have been available but in short supply.

Identifying the Virus

Being aware of it as a Virus Recognizing the Virus major distinctions between SARS and the current outbreak is the speed at which it was reported and how quickly researchers recognized it. On the 31st day of December in 2019, three weeks later than the initial incident, China told the World Health Organization about the new virus. 7 January was when they identified the virus responsible for the outbreak. This was as quick as any advanced country could have discovered it.

Genome sequencing can have a major impact-it assisting numerous countries in developing testing for viruses early and studying the virus. Following SARS, the virus was kept secret by China. The first time the disease was identified was in February 2003. However, at the time, five people had already died, and 300 had been ill from the virus in the Guangdong province in China. It wasn't that long after the initial SARS outbreak, American and Canadian scientists discovered that they had sequenced the genome, which is believed to be the cause of the virus. Health officials had struggled with the lack of information about the nature of the virus before 2003.

China has also done things differently this time. Beijing could study the genome and teach other nations about the concept. However, there are concerns about how transparent China is. Some worry that the scale of the problem could be more extensive than public figures suggest. Some coronavirus strains are not fatal. Those which are only found in human beings, like the common cold, are usually thought to be not reliable. However, the coronavirus that poses a risk of the pandemic is found in animals because the viruses were not present in humans before it was discovered that there isn't any obvious immunity in humans against these viruses.

CHAPTER 2

EVOLUTION AND IDENTIFICATION

The coronavirus, discovered at the end of the year, was from an animal to a human living in Wuhan, China. Within weeks, Wuhan has drawn enormous attention from scientists, the media, and the world community. The disease spreads quickly, and we are now aware of the new virus. The scientific community has been able to identify it as unable to comprehend everything at the start of 2020 by swabbing it to identify it and making the diagnostic test.

With each new outbreak, there are still many unanswered questions to be resolved as the disease advances, and researchers continue to develop more understanding of the nature of the disease. We'll attempt to inform you of the most important condition and information about epidemics in this episode. This week, the World Health Organization launched a strategy to combat the coronavirus that it has declared as an "international public health emergency" as the first individual within the U.S. with a confirmed infection from the hospital was discharged.

With more than 30000 verified cases reported in China, the World Health Organization, the covid-19 disease has claimed the lives of over 600 people. The virus has affected travel worldwide and caused governments and other agencies to adopt drastic steps to stop the spread of the virus across the globe, ranging from mass quarantines to evacuations. The Centres for Disease Control and Prevention stated that the virus isn't currently spread beyond those close to returning Wuhan travellers in China and the U.S.

Researchers are trying to comprehend the new threat and warn the public about current health initiatives that could lead to the development of a vaccine, including how the disease changes and transfers from one person to another. Specialists in infectious diseases at the Fred Hutchinson Cancer Research Centre, including Professor Dr Trevor Bedford, are the scientists at the forefront of this research. Bedford is a computational biologist studying how viruses develop and propagate and is currently gaining details about Covid-19 to help fight against this emerging respiratory virus.

As he researched the spread of the viral disease, Bedford presented what he's discovered to the media through interviews and the open-source platform that monitors the viral evolution in real-time that his staff has developed. Here are some examples of what Bedford and his colleagues have learned thus far, as well as the important questions they're still trying to answer:

- How can you minimize the risk of getting an infection?
- Signs

What are the most important things doctors and health professionals need to be aware of? Bedford's and other analyses on the DNA sequences of a few early human infections revealed that the virus showed a shocking lack of genetic diversity from one person to the next when it first showed up. The first issue was that there was not enough evidence to establish the meaning of this—did the virus continue to spread from humans to animals, or, even more importantly, was the virus rapidly spreading within humans following an initial animal leap? "DNA cannot separate these two cases." Only the animal in the reservoir can obtain epidemiological information or DNA. The process of determining this will be the primary goal of epidemiology for all.

I believe we're amid the possibility of a pandemic if it's not immediately implemented, "Bedford told STAT News on 27 January. However, Bedford warned that it's difficult to know how serious a Covid-19 outbreak could be. This kind of work done by Bedford and other trackers of viruses is possible because of the speedy genetic sequencing of those infected, which was impossible or possible not so long back—and an effort by all of us to communicate this genetic information with researchers around the globe freely.

In essence, just a week after the announcement that there's this brand new virus, the outstanding Chinese scientists have created discovered a genome for the virus that has never been observed. This first genome was a boon for researchers who wanted to develop quick tests to verify cases. The following genomes are extremely useful in understanding the basic epidemiological problems. "Adding some of the major samples could alter the narrative dramatically because of the rapid change in the character of the illness.

With access to more genetic sequences of more affected people, team members from Bedford and Nextstrain published a blog post on their site in January. 30 that they believe the lower rate of mutation for the illness is due to the process of the spread from unidentified species to humans in November or in the early days of December 2019 following its initial spike. The team also noted in their January. 30 update: Although the virus has begun to pick up new mutations when it is spread among people, this kind of virus is naturally able to do these mutations do not seem to be linked to any changes in the behavior in the viral. The new virus appears not to have the potential to harm people who have confirmed cases as its coronavirus predecessor, SARS. Still, data are not sufficient to draw definitive conclusions.

Bedford and co-workers explain their most recent findings on Covid-19 spread and its evolution across the globe. The map shows the amount and locations of the viral sequences they analyse in the course of the reach of China from patients around the world. In addition, a new analysis on the initial 425 individuals infected by a team of researchers based within China within the New England Journal of Medicine on 29 January. They discovered that it could take up to five days for someone diagnosed to experience symptoms after their first infection with the virus.

CHAPTER 3

REPORTED CASES ALL OVER THE WORLD

In December mid-December, the initial cases of coronavirus were confirmed in Wuhan. There have been confirmed coronavirus cases that have grown exponentially, and the infections have been detected across the globe. The hospitals located in Wuhan are already overcrowded, with hundreds of emergency medical professionals being sent to the area to assist. Two new hospitals are being built in the suburbs of the town, devoted to treating the disease.

The city's officials said over 4000 Wuhan residents lived overseas on 27 January. Wuhan's Wuhan Culture and Tourism office stated that after the lockdown was declared, all tours were cancelled; however, groups who left before the date had begun to return to the area slowly. More than 12 nations have been notified of Wuhan virus cases, and authorities struggle to stop spreading the disease.

More than 100 people have died due to a coronavirus epidemic in Wuhan, China, and over 4,600 people from 17 countries were afflicted. The virus, characterized as pneumonia and fevers, is believed to have originated from an unclean market in Wuhan, a city of 11 million people located in Hubei province in China. Authorities put Wuhan under quarantine on the morning of 23 January. They also stopped all public transport, including city buses, trains, and ferry services. The quarantine order will prohibit trains or buses from leaving or entering the city and stop every plane in the Wuhan airport. The Guardian reported that Wuhan authorities also began the following day with a ban on the travel of cars.

Huanggang City (home to around 7.5 million residents) was also shut up this week after authorities shut down train stations. 10 additional cities-Chibi, Enshi, Ezhou, Zhejiang, Chibi, Enshi, Ezhou, Huangshi, Suizhou, Qianjjiang, Xianning, Xiantao, Yichang, and

Zhejiang been following suit and imposed their travel restrictions for the following day. There are cities in Xiangyang, Jingmen, Xiaogan, and Dangyang were also quarantined at the time of this writing on Monday.

Wuhan is the fifth largest city in China and covers 3200 square miles. Contrastingly the city of New York, there are around 8 million residents within New York City—almost 3 million less than Wuhan. The town is split into three areas: Hankou, Wuchang, and Hanyang, with the rivers flowing through the middle. A majority of residents reside in one district but live in another section, which is why the travel ban between sections can disrupt the normal workings of the local community. According to the local authorities, it is no longer possible for people to leave Wuhan without the need for a "special reason," according to the local authorities.

In the meantime, officials from Huanggang demanded the closing of internet cafes and cinemas and advised people not to be allowed to go out of the town unless there are exceptional reasons, Reuters said. Trains and long-distance buses to the city are stopped. The city nearby, Ezhou, has also closed its train stations. In addition, buses in two smaller townships, Chibi and Zhejiang, were suspended. The quarantines were part of the celebrations of Lunar New Year, which started on a Saturday. The holiday is typically filled with the nation's buses, trains, bridges, ferries, and bridges with people from 3 billion who go home to visit their families. However, the Chinese government hases.

Several nations across Asia have increased airport screening and warned travellers not to travel to China. The neighbouring country of Mongolia has imposed strict restrictions on visitors traveling into the country to China's north. Indonesia and the Philippines have A total of a hundred people who have reported cases across the globe. The majority of these 14 are discovered in Thailand, the most popular tourist destination for Chinese tourists. Countries with colder climates are more likely to be affected in the future because the coronavirus thrives in colder climates and will not reproduce in hot, warm regions. In a case from Illinois, The Centres for Disease Control and Prevention announced the first instance of coronavirus transmission between humans within the U.S. The transmission was between two spouses, who kept in touch. The wife, an older woman who had travelled in Wuhan, China, was diagnosed in Wuhan, China. She was diagnosed with the disease. The husband lived in his 60s in Chicago, suffers from health issues, and does not travel to China. The risk for the general population in Illinois is still very low, "state health officials emphasized." They stated that they don't believe that the virus can spread widely to communities and are trying to ensure that health professionals are protected at the location where the patient is cared for. On Thursday evening, officials from the State Department released a" Do not Fly "advisory for China and its most severe warning. This Level 4 warning was already in place for the central area of the outbreak, Wuhan. The warning also recommended Americans get off commercial flights from China. The coronavirus is being investigated for 165 individuals in the United States. Of these, 68 were negative, while six tested positive. The tests of the remaining people are either in the process of being sent or have been reported in the pipeline.

Twenty American airports monitor travellers for signs of illness. They also give corona-virus signs to travellers returning from China with education documents. Many flights to China are being stopped by airlines around the world- United, Delta, American Airlines, British Airways, Air Seoul, Lion Air, Lufthansa Group, Cathay Pacific, Finnair, Air Asia, Air India, Air Canada, All Nippon Airways, Asiana Airlines, and Korean Air.

The US government charters a plane from Wuhan, China, to evacuate more than 196 Americans. The evacuees were checked and monitored before and during their flight to check for signs of disease. The passengers have been placed in the voluntary three-day quarantine after arriving in California. They will be provided surveillance for the virus as per the Centres for Disease Control and Prevention.

Though most reported cases outside of China are linked directly to Wuhan, there are signs that this virus may be beginning to spread to other countries. Three new cases have been reported in Germany, and the first human-to-human transmission to occur in Europe. Many countries have recommended avoiding visiting China because of the current epidemic. It is said that the US Base for Disease Regulator and Prevention (CDC) has issued a Level 3 advisory which advises against any "non-essential travel"—the highest level of alert on a scale from 1-to-3. However, there is no indication that the White House has denied reports of plans to pull all US-China flights.

With most of China experiencing cold weather suitable for the coronavirus and the ongoing doubts about how contagious the virus is, experts predict that the number of cases will remain on the rise for several weeks. Zhong Nanshan, one of the most renowned experts in the breathing of China and a hero in the war of 2003 against SARS, predicted the peak to be spotted within 10 to 14 days. It's difficult to pinpoint the time when the disease will strike. However, it is likely to reach the top in just one week or approximately 10 days, after which there won't be any massive increases.

However, others have cautioned that even though the Hubei outbreak could reach its peak within the next few weeks, other Chinese megacities could experience self-sustaining diseases that propagate the pathogen across the nation and the globe. An Australian laboratory was one of the very first laboratories outside China to discover an infection called COVID-19 using samples of patients. This will "provide important details to foreign specialist laboratories to combat the disease. We have developed epidemic curves that will last until August 2020 for the four major city clusters, including Chongqing Shanghai-Guangzhou, Shenzhen, and Beijing. Chongqing is expected to be the most affected due to its large population and the highest amount of traffic, paired with Wuhan.

Ecuador

On 26 January, Ecuador was among the first countries other than Mainland China to announce a suspected coronavirus infection. The Chinese resident of 49 years old came on the island of Hong Kong and showed symptoms of the illness. The Ministry of Health of Ecuador confirmed the case on 5 February; the coronavirus case was positive.

Botswana

In Botswana, five cases suspected of coronavirus infections have been confirmed. Each of them has been tested positive for the disease authorized by the Botswana officials on 5 February. On 30 January, the first corona case reported for coronavirus Botswana was reported as coronavirus, according to the Ministry of Health and Wellness, announced on 31 January. The suspect was brought in from China via the Ethiopian Airways flight, investigated, and isolated.

Czech Republic

By 4 February, 48 people were tested for the coronavirus, a novel type, and all tested positive, which the Czech Ministry of Health has confirmed. Respin Group, a Czech-based nanofibre technology company, has announced that it is working on a brand-new face mask that may reduce the spread of the coronavirus.

Namibia

On 1 February, Namibia Broadcasting Corporation (NBC) reported that a 30-year-old female who has symptoms similar to those associated with the coronavirus is being monitored in the hospital of Swakopmund, Namibia. The woman had been to Melbourne, Australia, and arrived at the international airport in Hosea Kutako. He observed that their return flight had Chinese passengers wearing masks and coughing. It was reported that the Namibia Ministry of Health said the details concerning the suspect incident NBC added. According to the Namibian Health Minister, Health announced on the 03rd of February that the suspected case had been confirmed to be positive.

Peru

The Peruvian Ministry of Health reported in its latest update of 3 February that there were no confirmed coronavirus cases in the region. The Ministry announced last week that the four suspected were negative for coronavirus.

Maldives

The Maldives striving to stop measles witnessed an individual who came via Xiamen, China, on 30 January. This was the first known coronavirus case. Six additional instances of Maldivians who had travelled to China were then discovered. The Ministry of Health of Maldives confirmed on 3 February that all cases tested positive for the virus.

Myanmar

The Chinese traveller's initial suspected coronavirus in Myanmar was reported on 31 January. The patient was from Guangzhou and took the flight of China Southern Airlines in Yangon. Of the 78 passengers the plane carried, only two were allowed to exit the aircraft, and the rest 76 were not allowed to exit, Anadolu Agency reported. But Myanmar said that the suspected case has been tested for the virus and found positive.

Ivory Coast (Cote d'Ivoire)

It was reported that the Ivory Coast confirmed one suspected corona virus-related infection on 26 January 2020. The patient, a 34-year-old female student, arrived to the Ivory Coast from Beijing to Abidjan. She was put in solitary confinement and was healthy throughout the observation period. The tests on her samples were positive for coronavirus authorities announced.

Ethiopia

It was discovered that four persons suspected of contracting the coronavirus and isolated in Addis Abeba were negative for the virus. Four of the students are studying in Wuhan City Universities.

Kenya

30 January 2020 Kenya announced the first confirmed case of coronavirus infection been confirmed to be negative. The patient was one of the Guangzhou travellers exhibiting symptoms of the disease. It was first announced on 28 January 2020. Upon arrival, the patient was initially placed in isolation in Jomo Kenyatta International Airport and later separated at the Kenyatta Hospital's Infectious Disease Unit. The tests revealed that the patient had a common cold but not a coronavirus infection.

Austria

Seven Austrians who arrived from China and were quarantined in the Hygiene Centre Vienna on 4 February were uninfected with coronavirus. On 2 February, the seven came to Austria and were late was administered to prevent the spread of the virus.

Mexico

Seven cases of suspected coronavirus were recorded within City, Mexico, all of which were negative on 27 January. The suspect cases comprised an older man aged 42 who was in Wuhan recently, one woman who was 37 years old, and a girl aged two who were in contact with the man. They receive medical care for respiratory illnesses as well. On Jalisco 20, January, three cases were recorded.

New Zealand

Tested positive on 31 February, the first case of reported confirmation by New Zealand. The doctor Ashley Bloomfield, the Director-General of Health, revealed the test results on 1 February. The person has contracted the disease and was placed in Auckland City Hospital in solitary confinement.

Cyprus

According to Cyprus News, a man from China who was accused of contracting coronavirus infection was tested positive on 2 February 2020. The patient was placed under observation at Nicosia's General Hospital of Nicosia on 31 January, following the onset of signs of illness.

Croatia

In the report by Total Croatia News, a man being held in isolation in the Split KBC hospital due to showing signs of coronavirus infection was found to be uninfected on 3 February. It was thought that he had contracted the virus after visiting China in the past on 2 February.

Switzerland

According to SWI, 28 January was when two cases suspected of coronavirus infection were confirmed negative. The two cases were approved on 27 January and were placed in solitary confinement in Zürich's Triemli hospital. The patients had been to China and had returned with symptoms of infection.

Greece

The Greek City Times reported that a sixty-year-old man believed suffering from coronavirus was negative for the illness. The man was put in quarantine by the General Hospital of AHEPA University.

Denmark

Denmark confirms that, as of 4 February, all patients tested for coronavirus were positive. The most recent testing was on passengers arriving at Wuhan to Roskilde Airport. A few days ago, a Danish woman returning from Wuhan with symptoms of infection was examined and isolated by the Aarhus University Hospital. The test was confirmed to be negative.

Ireland

Ireland believed that a person was to Wuhan infected by the coronavirus. They admitted the patient at the Royal Victoria Hospital, but the health department declared that tests were not positive The BBC published on 25 January.

On 31 January, World Health Organization identified 13 countries in Africa's continent, Africa, at risk of corona virus-related infections. These countries include Algeria, Angola, Cote d'Ivoire, Angola, the DRC, Ethiopia, Ghana, Kenya, Mauritius, Nigeria, South Africa, Tanzania, Uganda, and Zambia. They either have direct connections with China or manage the flow of many trips to China. Screening programs for active travellers were introduced at all countries' airports.

CHAPTER 4

57

OMS GLOBAL HEALTH EMERGENCY

In the absence of any indication that a coronavirus outbreak is diminishing, virologists are scouring worldwide to obtain the virus' physical samples. We are working on plans to test the effectiveness of vaccines and drugs, develop animal models of the disease, and study concerns regarding the virus's nature, including the ways it propagates. When we first heard of the outbreak, virologists began contacting people to access isolates. The epidemic's epicentre was the first lab to isolate and study the virus, dubbed Covid-19, located in Wuhan, China. A team headed by virologist Zheng-Li Shi at the Wuhan Institute of Virology isolated the virus from a 49-year older woman who began experiencing symptoms on 23 December before falling into a critical state. Shi's team discovered that the virus could destroy cultured human cells and infect them via the same molecular receptors as another coronavirus, the one that triggers SARS (severe acute respiratory syndrome). On 28 January, a laboratory in Australia confirmed that they had taken virus samples from an infected person returning from China. The team was preparing to share its findings with other researchers. The laboratories located in France, Germany, and Hong Kong are also analysing and plan to share samples of the virus they have collected from local patients they've managed.

Yet, a news-gathering held in Geneva at the World Health Organization declared the coronavirus as an emergency in public health that is of international concern. This is only the sixth time a crisis has been made, with previous examples being the Democratic Republic of Congo Ebola outbreak and Zika virus. By attempting to spread across the world, it is believed that the WHO can make the declaration for "extraordinary events" that present the risk of public health. This move reversed the WHO's decision to delay such announcements a week before. Since then, other countries and those of the United States have seen thousands of new cases of China and evidence of transmission from human to human. This has led to reconsideration from the committee on the emergency of W.H.O.

The announcement "is not a vote of mistrust in China." The W.H.O., on the contrary, appears to be believing that China can manage the spread. The announcement is made because of fears that the coronavirus may infect countries with weak health systems, where it could spread to the entire world, infecting many millions and causing the death of thousands.

The State Department warned travellers to beware of China completely following the announcement. The spokesperson of China's foreign ministry, Hua Chunying, stated that "the country is fully confident and able to win the fight against this epidemic." In a statement posted on its website, China will continue to work with W.H.O. and other countries to protect the public's health.

This announcement about the W.H.O. officially referred to as "an international public health emergency" is not subject to legal force. The department is overseen by an annual gathering attended by each of the U.N. health ministers. Their role is only to give instructions. The government will make its own decisions about how it can defend itself.

To Americans worried about their overall health, the best recommendation is to adhere to an effective flu season routine that includes frequent washing your hands, covering any coughs, and staying up-to-date with new CDC information. The CDC doesn't recommend wearing a face mask to prevent the coronavirus. We conclude that there is no immediate threat to the American population.

It is believed that the Illinois infection is the 6th outbreak of the coronavirus across the USA. The WHO deliberated over two weeks before deciding not to announce an emergency. However, individuals from Germany, Japan, Taiwan, Vietnam, and the United States are now infected by the coronavirus and have not visited China. The coronavirus of the new era is in the same family as SARS and the common cold.

Uncertainty arises from this human-to-human transmission occurring outside of China. Writing the novel, coronavirus has infected more than 7,700 individuals, and 170 people have died. More than 90 % of all deaths of those cases occurred in China. 20 % of the cases have been thought to be grave, while only 2 percent of them have resulted in death, as per the World health organization. The mortality rate for the most recent coronavirus is predicted to decrease because more infections are detected since the illest people are more likely to seek medical attention.

Emergency systems "just instructions. The government and private businesses "may or not be able to follow it." But, declarations of emergencies suggest a crucial emergency for the world's most prestigious medical advisory panel. The decision has been endorsed by many experts in the field of science. The crisis in public health "allows them to rely further on the role of global leadership for governments and the private sector."

The primary goal is to understand how the virus spreads, whether in hospitals or clinics or other settings, which ages and genders or jobs are most at risk, how sick, and which factors can be the most dangerous. But Amir Attaran, a law and epidemiology professor at the University of Ottawa and a frequent critic of W.H.O., called the announcement "inexcusably late." The reason for the committee's decision that it didn't have sufficient science-based evidence for declaring an emergency earlier this month was "balderdash," he said. SARS, Ebola, and Zika plague W.H.O. because of the same reasons which have destroyed its scientific expertise, "he said. Borders are shut, and planes have been grounded. ships docked like W.H.O. are quietly dithers about whether it is appropriate to announce the crisis. "Things have dramatically taken over them, showing their futility yet again," he said.

It is always a difficult decision to make. The closure of borders and cancellations of flights can cause suffering for millions of people close to the epicentre and a massive disruption to the economy. Food and medication supply can be depleted in extreme conditions

Experts from The W.H.O., however, have repeatedly and lavishly praised the response from China as violent and incredibly violent. In less than two weeks, the country has constructed two hospitals to care for patients suffering from the coronavirus. Chinese researchers have put the genetic signature of the coronavirus in libraries accessible to the public, which significantly accelerated the development of diagnostic tests and vaccines. The Chinese authorities fenced off the cities at the epicentre of the disease, Hubei Province, stranding more than 50 million people during the peak of New Year's celebrations-something that very few other nations could have made.

It is still to be determined how long this massive cordon will be successful. Five million people had the chance to escape Wuhan, where the outbreak first began before the city shut down its bus and train airports and stations. The Chinese Government has established a new standard for responding to the outbreak. Many countries should be happy that only 98 of almost 10,000 cases reported thus to date have occurred beyond the boundaries of China, the official stated.

Despite the state of emergency and how it is, the State Department advises Americans to avoid China; however, the W.H.O. opposes restrictions on travel and trade in China. According to the head of the agency's emergency committee

Other countries have implemented a variety of those measures against China. This doesn't mean that there weren't some mistakes. Last week, the W.H.O. classified its risk assessment of outbreaks by describing it as "moderate" when it should have used "high." The error was later added to the report as the footnote. U.S. researchers have written about the sporadic epidemiological information that comes from China. The W.H.O., too, does not share information with Taiwan that currently has eight patients suffering from the coronavirus, because Taiwan is not an official participant in the UN.

The company "doesn't want any of its primary customers to be up in arms. China holds the political influence that many other countries do not have. But, in addition to its consequences, the disease is accelerating. On Friday, China announced that another 43 people had died of the illness, taking up 213. There are not yet been any deaths outside of China.

Russia closed a significant portion of its 2,600-mile border with China and stopped all trains, except regular trains connecting Moscow and Peking. Many airlines, such as British Airways, stopped flying there, while others cut their operations significantly. Certain medical experts in China have criticized the government's response and argued that the local authorities should have instituted more strict travel restrictions before the disease spreads from Wuhan. China is now experiencing confirmed cases in every province and zone.

Some have claimed that local authorities were silent about the extent of the disease, initially claiming there was no evidence of transmission between individuals outside Wuhan and then revealing the truth following Hong Kong press reports. The severity of the disease became clear Wuhan's mayor announced his resignation on Monday.

A group of the W.H.O. was allowed to visit Wuhan for just one day of rain. The official stated that the visit was not meant to render judgment. Every step is done in a spirit of determination and good practice to threes assessment. It is essential to understand the huge scope and depth of the initiative. "After the trip, China agreed to allow W.H.O.-coordinated experts from around the world to collaborate with Chinese researchers to combat the spread of the disease within this area. A team that will be part of the team is put together from members of the C.D.C. From its inception at the end of 2005, it has been a long time since the W.H.O. has made only five emergency declarations to address the outbreak of flu as well as for the 2014 polio resurgence in the case of West African Ebola epidemic during that year; for the Zika virus was able to erupt in 2016, and for an Ebola spread that occurred in Congo Democratic Republic of Congo last year.

It has also taken vital steps, including regular communication with WHO and strong multi-sector strategies to prevent further spread. In the provinces and other cities, they have also implemented measures to improve public health by researching the spread and severity of the virus and sharing information and biological content. China has also agreed to collaborate with other countries that need assistance. The actions China has taken are beneficial for China and the global community. The Committee acknowledged WHO and its partners as having an important player.

The Committee also acknowledged that many are still unsolved. Still, cases are now being identified within five WHO regions in less than a month, and the human-to-human transmission has been reported out of Wuhan and outside of China.

The Committee affirms that it is feasible to limit the spread of the virus when countries implement efficient measures to detect illness early, identify and treat cases, track interactions, and encourage risk-sensitive social distancing. It is crucial to remember that, as the issue continues to change in the future, the strategic objectives and strategies to stop and slow the spread of infection will also change. The Committee determined that the situation has now met global public health emergency requirements. They provided the following suggestions to be used as temporary Recommendations.

The Committee stressed that a statement from a PHEIC is to be taken as a gesture of respect and support for China and its people, and China's actions at the frontlines of this epidemic, with the utmost transparency and, it's to be hoped, improvement. In keeping with the need to unite the world, the Committee recognized the need for an international coordination effort to increase the preparedness of other regions of the globe that could require more support.

The Committee applauded the upcoming trip to China, including local and national experts from the WHO. The mission will analyze and aid efforts to study the origins of the disease and the clinical and severity that the illness is causing, the level of human-to-human transmission within the community and health facilities, and efforts to manage the outbreak. The task will supply the world community with the information needed to understand the issue and its consequences and will aid in sharing knowledge and efficient actions.

The Committee wanted to emphasize the importance of investigating the potential source, including excluding transmission by secret and providing the steps to manage risk. The Committee stressed the importance of more thorough surveillance of non-Hubei regions, such as genomic sequencing of pathogens, to determine if the local transmission cycle occurs.

The World Health Organization should continue to use its specialist networks worldwide to identify the best method to combat the spread of the disease globally. WHO should offer greater preparation and support for a response, particularly in areas and countries with high vulnerability. It is essential to establish measures to promote rapid growth and accessibility for countries with low and middle incomes to future vaccines, antiviral medicine, and other treatments.

WHO must continue to provide the operational and technical support required to combat this outbreak, in conjunction with its vast network of partners and other organizations, to implement a strong strategy for communicating risk and allow scientific research and advances regarding this unique coronavirus to continue.

The WHO is expected to continue investigating the feasibility of creating an intermediate level of warning that can distinguish between the two possibilities of PHEIC or not so that discussions about the IHR text don't need to be revisited (2005).

The WHO will evaluate the situation consistently as needed and then amend its recommendations based on research. The Committee is not proposing any travel restrictions or trade based on the available information. The Director-General announced that the outbreak of Covid-19 was a PHEIC, accepted the Committee's recommendations, and issued this recommendation as Temporary Recommendations within the IHR.

To the People's Republic of China:

Create a comprehensive risk communication plan to inform the people regularly about the severity of the outbreak, the public's security and prevention measures, and the steps to stop it.

- Improve public health programs to stop the current epidemic.

* Ensure stability in the health system and secure healthcare professionals.

- Increase the monitoring of and success case-finding across China.

* Collaborate with WHO and its partners on studies that identify the origins and the evolution of the disease and the steps to control it.

* Take advantage of the relevant human case details.

* Continue to look for the zoonotic cause of the infection when it is available and, in particular, the possibility of spread with WHO;

* Conduct the exit screen at all international ports and airports to ensure prompt detection to evaluate further and treat patients while minimizing interference with international travel.

To all nations:

* A greater number of foreign-exported cases are anticipated in any area. Every country should be prepared for the possibility of containment by ensuring active surveillance, early detection, the isolation of patients, and their management monitoring of communication and prevention of the spread of Covid-19 and complete sharing of data with the World Health Organization. Professional guidance is available on the WHO website.

The countries are reminded that the IHR legally binds them to share data with the WHO.

* Any detection of the Covid-19 virus in animals (including details about the species, diagnostic tests, and other pertinent epidemiological data) must be reported as a new illness to the World Organization for Animal Health (OIE).

* The countries should put a special emphasis on reducing the risk of human infections, and prevent secondary transmission and spread across the globe, and contribute to international responses through multi-sector collaboration with active engagement in increasing awareness of diseases and viruses and advancing research.

* The Committee has not proposed any travel restrictions or trade based upon the most current information available.

* The countries must be required to inform the WHO as per the IHR of any actions taken to travel. States are advised against activities that promote prejudice or stigma, as per The IHR's Article 3 Principles.

* Given the rapid change in this situation, The Committee asked the Director-General to give further direction regarding these issues and, if required to make case-by-case suggestions.

To the international community:

* Since this is a brand-new coronavirus and has been proven previously that coronaviruses like this require a lot of efforts to permit regular information sharing and research, the international world will display unity and cooperation by supporting each one another in identifying the cause of this new coronavirus as per Article 44 of the IHR (2005).

• Help countries with low and middle incomes to deal with this situation and increase the availability of diagnostics, treatments, and vaccines.

By Art. 43, IHR States Parties that adopt other health-related measures which significantly hinder international travel (refusal to allow entry or deportation for longer than 24 hours for international travellers, luggage, containers, cargo transport, goods, and similar) must submit to the WHO an explanation and justification to protect public health in the first 48 hours after their arrival. WHO will examine the rationale and ask the country to reconsider its decisions. WHO is obliged to provide information on interventions and their reasons in other State Parties. The health department of the UN stated that the decision was made to safeguard countries that have "weaker health systems," however, the WHO also said that there was no justification for measures that could interfere with trade and travel between countries.

CHAPTER 5

PREVENTIVE MEASURES BY COUNTRIES

Researchers and health professionals worldwide are working to stop the spreading of the fatal virus discovered in December in Wuhan, the Chinese town of Wuhan. The coronavirus is a new strain already infected by thousands of people and can trigger respiratory illness. The death toll stands at 213 and is expected to increase over time. The World Health Organization (WHO) declared a "public health emergency of international concern" by World Health Organization (WHO) on 30 January. It alerted its issues for situations that present an imminent threat to multiple nations and require an international response.

How many people are the Virus able to infect?

It is believed that the Chinese authorities have retreated to cities that are at the heart of the outbreak. Researchers have been quick to share data on the virus with researchers at the World Health Organization and with researchers. However, the number of cases has increased, and over 9,000 cases have risen within the last day, predominantly in China. This has led to an estimate that the virus may be affecting 39,000 of the 30 million people who live throughout Wuhan. Wuhan region. It appears that the virus escaped the control of China and spread too widely rapidly for it to be managed.

In the ideal situation, there is a lower chance of getting affected because the effects of the prevention measures will begin to show, according to University of Hong Kong epidemiologist Ben Cowling. It's too early to determine whether efforts are effective to protect men from infection and the widespread use of face masks. He adds that the incubation time of the virus, up to 14 days, is more than most prevention measures in place.

According to a different model of prediction, around 190,000 people might be sick within Wuhan in the event of a catastrophe. Scientists are especially concerned about the emergence of new outbreaks outside of China. The virus is already spreading in tiny, scattered clusters across Vietnam, Japan, Germany, and the U.S., but officials have isolated affected individuals. On 30 January, fewer than 100 cases were confirmed outside of China.

Is the Virus Here to Stay?

It's believed to be normal for a virus to circulate throughout a population. There are many nations where the virus that causes influenza and chickenpox are widespread, but they can be controlled by vaccination and keeping individuals at home when sick.

The biggest question is whether coronavirus is still around to stay. If attempts to eradicate the virus fail, then there's a high chance it will eventually become widely spread. It could be the case, just like with the flu, that deaths happen every year due to the spread of the virus until a vaccine can be developed. If those suffering from the virus but don't have symptoms are infected, it becomes more difficult to stop its spread, and it is more likely to make the virus an endemic disease for them.

Certain cases of people infected with no symptoms have occurred, and it's unclear if these asymptomatic or light cases can be considered normal and the degree of contagiousness. "Probably we are looking at a virus that will be with us for a long time, possibly forever," Mackay declares.

Asymptomatic cases distinguish the new virus from the coronavirus that causes serious acute respiratory symptoms (SARS). The virus was a worldwide outbreak in 2002-03, but it usually did not spread until people became sick enough to require hospitalization. Once seizures were controlled within hospitals, SARS could be handled. There's no evidence to suggest that the virus isn't spreading in humans, claims Mackay.

Suppose the measures to control the outbreak are successful and transmission decreases to the point where no greater than one gets infected per person infected. In that case, the current outbreak might be a temporary occurrence, as Cowling suggests.

Is the Virus Likely To Change?

Certain researchers are worried that the pathogen may change as China's coronavirus spreads to make it possible to be more easily applied or increase the likelihood of causing illness among children. The virus is currently causing serious diseases and deaths, especially in the elderly, and pre-existing diseases like heart disease and diabetes. The newest victim to be identified thus far is a 36-year old Wuhan man with no known existing health issues.

Kristian Andersen Kristian Andersen, a Scripps Research infectious-disease expert in La Jolla, California, isn't worried about the virus becoming infective. He believes that viruses are constantly altering as part of their lifespan; however, these changes usually do not make them more dangerous or trigger severe illnesses. "I can't think of any cases of this having happened with pathogenic outbreaks," he adds.

Suppose viruses move between a host animal and another—which could be why the coronavirus currently started infecting humans. In that case, there could be some selection pressure within the new host to increase longevity. Still, it rarely is ever, if ever, an effect on the spread of the disease. Certain mutations harm the virus or are of no consequence. A study conducted in 2018 of SARS inside primate chambers revealed that the virus's virulence could be reduced by a mutation sustained through the epidemic of 2003.

Researchers have swapped hundreds of sequences derived from the most recent coronavirus strains. MacKay said that a constant amount of these samples would reveal genetic modifications as the disease grows. "If they change the sequence, viruses do not change behavior, and we need to see persistent or consistent virus change," MacKay says.

How Many People Will It Kill?

The mortality rate of a virus—the proportion of those infected who die it is hard to determine in the middle of an outbreak since reports are continually updated with the latest cases and deaths. The latest coronavirus has a mortality rate of 2 to 3 percent and 213 points so far of more than 10,000 cases. This is significantly less than SARS which claimed the lives of about 10% of the patients. The death rate reported for the coronavirus in the news will likely decrease as mild cases. Those who are symptomatic are discovered in the future, an expert in virology, Mark Harris at Leeds University, UK, told London's Science Media Centre.

There are no drugs that work to fight the virus at the present moment. Two HIV treatments that focus on a protein that assists in replicating coronaviruses are being investigated for a possible cure. Scientists have discovered numerous therapies targeting this function, and many intercontinental research groups are working with the serum.

The number of people who die will be contingent on how the health system in China handles a high number of cases. Placing patients on ventilators and drips can ensure that they get sufficient oxygen and fluids while the immune system within their body fights against the disease. China is currently building two clinics at Wuhan to treat people who are sick; however, if the infection is spread to other parts of the globe with fewer resources, for instance, African high-income regions, the health systems of these regions could fail, according to Sanjaya Senanayake expert in infectious diseases within Canberra's Australian National University.

The director-general of the WHO, Tedros Adhanom Ghebreyesus, stated that his primary reason for the announcement of an emergency in the world health system was the risk that the outbreak could be spread to countries that have weak health systems.

If SARS is spreading across the globe, the number of people dying could prove substantial. In the case of infectious disease, the current mortality rate of 2-3 percent is not as high as that of SARS but very high. The outbreak of influenza in 1918, also known as the Spanish flu, afflicted around half a billion people, one-third of the world's population. It also caused death to more than 2.5 percent of infected. Other reports suggested that up to 50 million people were killed. The case of the COVID-19 virus isn't likely to cause this kind of scenario since it is not known to cause death or infection to healthy people in their teens.

How Long Will It Take to Exploit a Serum?

A vaccine is one year away, at the very minimum. The coronavirus vaccine could keep the virus from spreading and prevent the spread of the disease. However, it takes some time before the vaccines are effective. The advancement of technology, new developments in genomics, and improved global collaboration have allowed researchers to develop at an unimaginable speed; the development of vaccines is a risky and costly procedure. Scientists typically need to begin from scratch each time a new outbreak occurs. Following 2003's SARS outbreak was reported, it took 20 months to develop the vaccine in place for trials on humans. (The vaccine was never required since it could contain the virus.) In 2015, following the Zika outbreak, experts had lowered the development timeframe for vaccines down to six months.

The researchers hope that the findings from previous outbreaks can reduce the timeframe. Scientists have already studied the coronavirus genome and have identified the crucial proteins for infection. National Institutes of Health scientists from Australia and at least 3 companies are currently working on vaccine candidates.

If they do not encounter any unexpected problems, A Phase 1 trial will likely be completed within three months. The experts cautioned that it could take months or even years to conduct thorough tests following preliminary trials that prove the vaccine's safety and efficiency. A vaccine can most likely be accessible to the general public within a year from today.

What happens if I'm on the road?

Traveling to China during this time could be dangerous. It's unclear how the virus could be spread or which individuals are at the greatest risk of getting a bad result. Hubei is being issued an alert for travel of Level 4 issued by The U.S. State Department, which signifies "do not fly" and is the highest alert level. For the remainder of China, a Level 3 alert is in effect. The greatest risk to travel to China is that China is currently under quarantine. The Chinese government has put in place strict travel bans and quarantines. If you must travel to China, where there have been reports of the virus, experts suggest wearing masks and washing your hands frequently, and staying clear of anyone sick.

Be aware that over-the-counter masks don't protect against airborne illnesses, and the shows won't work should the virus evolve and becomes airborne. In the United States, the CDC is continuously monitoring the condition. The CDC was investigating 165 cases on the 29th of January 2020. Four were upheld. Arizona, Washington, California, and Illinois are the states that have confirmed cases.

Should I Wear a Surgical Mask To Protect Myself?

If you suffer from an infection of the respiratory tract wearing a mask can assist in protecting the others around you from becoming sick by limiting the possibility of spreading the disease. If there's an outbreak wearing a mask for surgery could be able to protect you from infections within crowds. But, generally speaking, the surgical covers aren't tight-fitting enough to suck up every ounce of air that you breathe. The heavy-duty N95 respirators can be extremely uncomfortable. The experts recommend that you clean your hands throughout the day. Do not touch your face, and stay away from those who cough or cough.

The risk of getting infected within the United States with the latest coronavirus is a bit low for the average person to begin wearing an eye mask. If you're suffering from an illness that causes respiratory symptoms, wearing masks can reduce the risk of spreading the virus to others. "I've planned for a trip to China, and I'm wondering if I should take a trip?

I Have a Trip Planned to China; Should I Go?

Don't go. The state department has advised Americans not to visit China unless required. Suppose it's appropriate for tourists to travel and visit China. In that case, the C.D.C. suggests taking extra precautions to beware of contact with anyone who is sick and the animals and markets they are sold and refrain from eating raw or not cooked meat.

Anyone over 50 or with an existing health condition that could increase the risk of contracting an infection should speak with the health professional before taking a trip. In light of the situation and the difficulty in accessing medical treatment in China is likely to be difficult Federal officials have advised that new restrictions on travel, such as quarantine, maybe in place after returning. Many airline companies have cancelled their flights for China, and many travellers are in uncertainty as they search for flights to modify or revoke.

What are Health Authorities Doing to Contain the Virus?

It's no surprise that 2020 started the new decade in China by announcing an entirely new risk to the coronavirus (Covid-19). Human behavior and environmental influences caused over the last thirty years, to the development of more than 30 new infections ranging from rotavirus, which can cause infantile diarrhea and various other diseases, to Middle East respiratory coronavirus syndrome first recognized in 2012. The human population continues to increase, the demand for land for agriculture is growing, exposing livestock and people to diseases of the wildlife. Climate change also affects the number of animals, environmental numbers, the rapid flow of air traffic, the movement of people across different borders, and the conflict and political instability that creates the possibility that these new diseases are easily spreading all over the globe.

China implemented extreme measures to stop the people from leaving the affected areas; however, five million people remained in Wuhan in peace before the bans. On December 8, 2019, the Chinese government announced the deaths of one patient and 41 others admitted to hospitals with no cause in Wuhan, central China2, with an estimated total population of 10 million. It is also an important transport hub3. The Chinese government shut down an industry that sells seafood which sells live animals of exotic species for food, from the 1st of January in 2020, a mere months after the first cases were identified. Most of the 41 confirmed cases were determined to have connections to.

The public was also advised to wear masks to help prevent the virus from spreading. The two new facilities are being constructed for people suffering from coronavirus. The first hospital began operations on Monday. The governments of the globe have been screening the new

Chinese travellers in search of signs that indicate illness, as well as some of them, have taken it further by preventing individuals from China from getting into it. Many of the borders between China were shut down through Russia and Mongolia. Australia has stated that it will expel Wuhan citizens and quarantine them at Christmas Island for 14 days.

Chinese experts and international scientists led a group swiftly joining forces in a huge international and national collaboration effort. This comprised Shanghai Public Health Medical Centre and the Shanghai Public Health Medical Centre and Public Health School, Wuhan Central Hospital and the Chinese Centre for Disease Control and Prevention (CDC), Huazhong University of Science and Technology, and Wuhan University of Science and Technology, Wuhan Centre for Disease Control and Prevention and The National Institute for Communicable Disease Control and Prevention and the University of Sydney, Australia.

On January 10, 2020, the team had sequenced and released portions of sequences derived from a Wuhan patient with at least 70% genetic material resemblances to SARS (SARS) 5. The openness of divulging information about the sequence is essential in developing diagnostic tests and future treatments and vaccines to control the spread of the disease in case it spreads widely. The sequences were stored within GenBank (code MN908947 to access). Recent research suggests that the death rate for Covid-19 (2 deaths in 48 confirmed cases in the laboratory, which is 4.1 percent) could be lower than SARS. A knowledge of Covid-19's reservoir, pathogenesis, and the clinical spectrum also needs to be developed.

This latest disease by the Chinese government has been swift and decisive. This indicates a significant deviation from the public health policies, which led to the death of 774 people in the 2002 SARS epidemic, the spread of the virus to 37 different countries, and the loss of over US40 billion in six months. China has made great strides in its response to diseases in less than two years. First, a major shift in the attitude of the Chinese government towards public health has caused China to acknowledge that a new coronavirus is present quickly. The Chinese government didn't report the unusual new disease in the World Health Organization until 4 months after the first outbreak was reported due to a 2003 SARS outbreak.

The second was that the government took the lead in closing the market for fish in Wuhan, learning of the SARS outbreak, which ended when the palm civet consumed by people in China has been identified as the cause and was removed from the market.

The rapid growth of a global and national group has swiftly diagnosed the virus and released the virus's sequences to the general public in just a few days. On 24 March 2003, just five years after the first case was identified in November 2002, the first sequences of laboratory tests showed the existence of a new coronavirus was the reason for SARS. The 2002 SARS epidemic demonstrated the weaknesses of China's leading public health institution, the China CDC program. Nevertheless, once the epidemic ended, through the Field Epidemiology Training Program, the government prioritized improving CDC processes, improving public health monitoring and laboratory services, and the workforce-development program. There is no doubt that the increase in public health services and facilities will play a significant role in the fight against the Covid-19 outbreak currently in progress. Yet, a study conducted in 2012 highlighted the amazing improvement made in the China CDC since 2002, leading to quicker responses to emerging outbreaks and the overall quality of health services offered by the public increasing drastically from 47.4 percent to 76.6 percent.

China CDC has played a crucial role in improving the country's public health system. The agency also acknowledges that global diseases are likely to affect China, so it is actively exporting its knowledge to assist other developing countries to better prepare and react to new pathogen outbreaks. This includes active support for the 2013 outbreak in West Africa's Ebola virus. C.D.C. teams also aid in health-related investigations by the state of health and diseases, such as contact monitoring which ensures that any person who has come in contact with an affected person is warned of the risk and is monitored. This research will increase knowledge of the virus and prevent it from spreading. C.D.C. teams have also offered to send experts from general health and public safety to China to aid in the testing and efforts to contain the outbreak. The development of the Chinese Centre for Disease Control and Prevention was the turning point for regional response to epidemics. It is an important step and progress for security and diplomacy in the global health system.

Building Hospitals to provide Corona disease Care and Treatment

China has planned to open Dabie Mountain Regional Medical Centre Dabie Mountain Regional Medical Centre, a hospital with 1,000 beds, through the speed of its construction and to open it up to patients who have corona-related symptoms quarantine on the 29th of January. It's also developing a second hospital for quarantine named Leishenshan that will have as many as 1,500 beds within Wuhan.

A brand new hospital with 1,000 beds, known as Huoshenshan hospital, was completed in a mere ten days to provide better medical care and treatment for patients suffering from the coronavirus. The temporary hospital was officially opened on February 03 to accept patients.

China plans to transform 11 of the facilities located in Wuhan city of Wuhan, including gymnasiums exhibition centers and sports facilities, into temporary hospitals with more than 10,000 beds to treat patients suffering from mild ailments. Eight more sites that will be turned into hospitals were revealed. On February 3, the first three hospitals were transformed into hospitals, with 3400 beds to treat patients.

In addition, 20 mobile hospitals and 1400 nurses from across the nation were brought to Wuhan to help patients suffering from mild symptoms. Also, there was the building of an infected illness hospital located within Zhengzhou, Henan Province.

The biopharmaceutical business created two diagnostic kits for the coronavirus antigen that was discovered created by the Wuhan Institute of Virology of the Chinese Academy of Sciences. The virus can be detected within two hours or longer using an improved testing method developed at Wuhan University's Zhongnan Hospital, which has been said in the prompt start of treatment and improved recovery.

It is worth noting that the National Medical Products Administration also approved on the 26th of January two diagnostic kits and an instrument for testing developed by biopharmaceutical firms based in Hubei. In the meantime, efforts to develop vaccines are progressing by using two chemical compounds that are effective in limiting the activity of viruses which will aid in helping the new coronavirus speed up the development of drugs. Wuhan Jinyintan Hospital was the first hospital to use Kaletra (lopinavir or the ritonavir) as the treatment for HIV and AIDS for treating patients suffering from novel coronavirus and to be aware that it is completely safe. It is safe. Chinese Academy of Sciences has made available free and open access to Chinese researchers to the resources and services provided by the China Science and Technology Cloud (CSTC) to support their Covid-19 research. To facilitate collaboration with other researchers, researchers must have the ability to access high-performance computers, software, and other tools.

Baidu Research has allowed gene testing organizations, disease control centres, and research institutes to use LinearFold. Their RNA structure analysis algorithm will aid in understanding how viruses spread and screen chemicals within less than a minute, compared to about an hour before.

Why Africa Should Be Prepared

On the 20th of January, 2020, The Chinese government announced 136 new cases of the virus, which were reported to other cities in the country during the weekend and brought the number of confirmed cases to nearly 200 in the world (ref. 10). Infections with Covid-19 are now being reported in other countries of the region. A case of Covid-19-related infection in a 61-year-old Chinese visitor in Wuhan located in Bangkok was reported in Thailand on January 8th, 2011. On January 10, 2010, a patient of male age was confirmed as admitted to the hospital by officials from the Japanese Ministry of Health and was confirmed negative for the disease. They also confirmed probable cases to Hong Kong and Singapore.

The investigation of the models suggests that over 1,700 people might have been affected. The study, which included an overall confidence period of 95 percent, ranging between 427 and 4,471, was based on Wuhan's large international air traffic. This city is an important travel hub, as well as the duration of incubation for patients within Thailand in Thailand and Japan.

Because of the flight traffic and massive movement of people, the rapid spread of Covid-19 in Asia will be a major issue in Africa. The SARS disease was mostly spared from Africa in 2002, and only one case was reported within South Africa—a businessman traveling across the ocean to Hong Kong. However, as a result of the rapid growth of Chinese investments in Africa18, the number of flights between China and Africa has increased by over 600 percent in the last decade. For instance, Ethiopian Airlines, Africa's largest airline, currently is responsible for nearly 50% of Africa's annual 2,616 flights to China18.

Thus, African countries need to be vigilant and enhance their surveillance of public health and lab networks, coordinated by public health authorities in the country that is functional to prepare better to stop, detect and monitor any possible spreading of the disease across the continent swiftly. The efforts are being coordinated to cooperate between those of the Africa Centers for Disease Control and Prevention located in Addis Abeba in Ethiopia and China CDC to share information about people who may be sick. Traveling through China to Africa is also required to be coordinated.

China's willingness to provide rapid coverage and the identification of the Covid-19 virus as a novel and the swift sequence and the public distribution of the sequences is the dawn of a new day in global security of health and the international diplomacy of health. Furthermore, there is a chance that China CDC's sturdier networks will yield a massive benefit from public health investments in fighting the epidemic if it expands throughout China. This will also enhance global health protection because the worldwide healthcare chain can only be as robust as its weakest link; thus, a disease threat can easily be a threat anyplace.

List of Countries That Have Restricted or Banned Chinese Tourists or Visitors

On February 2nd, 2020 on February 2, 2020, the US published the highest-level travel advisories (level 4.) and advised its citizens not to travel to China. The US also urged US citizens living in China to travel whenever possible by commercial methods or to stay in their homes and avoid contact with others. On the 1st of February, 2020, Australia announced heightened border controls to stop transmission of the disease. Every passenger who arrives is subject to increased screening procedures, and, starting January 1, 2020, travellers who leave China are barred from entering the country. This includes Australian citizens and permanent residents, and members of their immediate families.

New Zealand imposed temporary travel restrictions for foreigners from China to New Zealand. The restrictions were imposed for 14 days and must be checked at least every 48 hours.

On February 3, 2020, Maldives announced new security precautions at the border that will limit the entry of passengers from China and China, except for Maldivian citizens or those who travelled through China. The Maldivians also were warned of non-essential travel to China and other countries afflicted by the virus.

Indonesia, Israel, Iraq, Italy, Honduras, El Salvador, Oman, Saudi Arabia, Russia, Japan, Vietnam, Singapore, and Pakistan are a few other countries that have placed travel restrictions on or cancelled direct flights for China, according to the BBC Reuters.

Fiscal Measures to Minimize Economic Impact: Liquidity Infusion and Tariff Cuts

The cuts in Coronavirus outbreaks could cause more harm to the global economy than the spread in 2003. SARS (Severe Acute Respiratory Syndrome) in 2003, because any recession in the Chinese economy won't cause waves, but rather ripples around the world, IHS Markit said Friday.

The virus has halted much of the world's second-largest economy, and its impact has been felt throughout industries. Coronavirus is likely to be more damaging to the world economy than in 2003's SARS outbreak. China was the 6th largest economy when it was hit by SARS and accounted for just 4.2 percent of the world's GDP. China currently is the second biggest economy worldwide, accounting for 16.3 percent of the world's GDP. Thus, any dip of the Chinese economy doesn't cause waves, but ripples that ripple all over the world, "IHS said in a statement on the outbreak of coronavirus.

In this instance, coronaviruses and the following measures will decrease the real global GDP by 0.4 percent in 2020. In contrast, the measures to contain it begin to take effect on 10 February, the effect on GDP globally will be less significant, resulting in 0.1 percent.

The negative effects of coronavirus on consumption by households are the most severe and are somewhat less in the industrial industry because factories are closed for the season during this period. But China's economic situation is more vulnerable in many ways than it was back in 2003, with both production and overall economic growth slowing, and the negative effects of the trade war between China and the US as well as China, "it said.

Since SARS and its impact on the global economy have become much greater than ever before, China's GDP has grown significantly.

Chinese slowdown in growth could be a significant stumbling block to global change. China has contributed 23 percent of world economic growth between 2002 and 2003. China is the main contributor to 38 percent of global growth in 2019, "IHS stated.

The People's Bank of China (PBOC) revealed strategies to carry the RMB1.2tn ($173bn) reverse purchase operations to ensure the availability of liquidity for the economy. Banks' liquidity amounts to RMB900bn ($129bn) greater than what was reported during the previous year at the same period. China is also expected to announce a reduction in tariffs on imports from countries such as the US to guarantee supplies in the wake of the current trade war between both countries.

Non-Fiscal Measures

The Chinese Trade Ministry ensures that sufficient stocks of pork, beef, and other essential food items, are kept in place to prevent shortages. As part of preventive security measures taken by several of the biggest and busiest international airports to stop coronavirus spread after the spread within Wuhan, China, many other countries took similar actions. Coronaviruses spread across 25 additional countries in just a month, which led to the closure of borders and a host of nations to declare health emergencies.

CDC Response

To fight this health problem to combat this issue, the federal government is in close collaboration with local, state, and tribal partners in addition to public health organizations. The public health approach is multi-layered to identify and reduce introductions of the virus in the United States to reduce the impact and spread of the virus. On January 7, 2020, CDC created a Covid-19 Incident Management Program. CDC began to activate the Emergency Operations Centre on January 21, 2020, to support covid-19.

CDC issued a revised health advisory for China on the 27th of January, 2020, which recommends that travellers stay clear of any non-essential travel within the entire country (Level 3 Health Notification).

The U.S. government has taken unprecedented measures to travel in response to the growing threat of the emerging coronavirus to public health. As of February 2nd in 2020, at 5 pm, the U.S. government has prohibited the entry of foreigners who have been within China for the last 14 days.

U.S. citizens, visitors, and family members of their immediate relatives who have visited Hubei Province and other areas of mainland China are allowed to enter the U.S. Still; they are required to undergo health screening and possibly isolation for up to 14 days. On February 1, 2020, the CDC issued the interim Health Alert Network (HAN) update that notified local and state health departments and health experts regarding this outbreak.

On January 30 the year 2020 CDC issued guidelines for the treatment of Covid-19 patients intended for healthcare professionals. CDC published guidelines on February 3rd, 2020, to assess the risk of various exposures to Covid-19 and help appropriately treat patients.

CDC is sending multidisciplinary teams into Oregon, Illinois, California, Arizona, and Wisconsin to assist hospitals, information gathering, and outreach divisions for safety. CDC developed a real-time Reverse transcription-polymerase Chain Reaction (rRT-PCR) test that can diagnose Covid-19 from clinical specimens in both respiratory and serum samples. CDC publicized the test protocol for the trial on 24 January of 2020. The CDC provided to those in the United States an Emergency Use Authorization (EUA) kit, food and Drugs Administration for their review on February 3, 2020. On February 4, 2020, it was announced that the FDA accepted the EUA. On the 5th of February, 2020, CDC testing kits were made available for purchase through the FDA's International Reagent Service External symbol from both international and domestic partners. After sequencing, CDC submitted the virus's entire genome from the reported cases within the United States to GenBank. CDC has created the Covid-19 virus as a cell-cultured virus which is needed for further research, including more study of genetic characterization. The virus grown on cells is being sent to the NIH BEI Tool symbol for the entire scientific community to utilize.

Delta Variant:

On the 27th of July, 2021, CDC issued updated guidelines on the necessity of an immediate increase in the coverage of COVID-19 and a suggestion for everyone living in areas of <u>high</u> or significant exposure to wear a mask when visiting public indoor spaces even if they're completely vaccination-free. CDC issued the new guidelines in response to a variety of concerning developments and the emergence of new data signalling.

A significant rise in the number of new cases reversed an ongoing decline from January 2021. In the weeks leading up to the release of our guidance, CDC saw a rapid and alarming rise in the rate of hospitalization and COVID-19 cases across the nation.

- In the latter part of June, the 7-day movement average of cases that were reported was approximately 12,000. On the 27th of July, the seven day movement average for cases climbed more than 60,000. The rate of cases looked like the rates of cases we'd seen before the vaccine became widely accessible.

Then, new evidence emerged that showed that it was evident that the Delta variation was much more contagious and was contributing to an increase in transmissibility when compared with other variants, including those who were vaccinated. This includes recently released information of CDC together with our partner in the public sector non-published surveillance data that will be available to the public in the next few weeks, data that is included in the CDC's revised science brief on COVID-19 vaccines, and Vaccination and ongoing investigations into outbreaks linked in this Delta variant.

Delta is currently the dominant type of virus that is currently prevalent within the United States. Here is an overview of the information CDC scientists have discovered regarding Delta. Delta variant. More details will be available once more data are released or made available in different formats.

1 SARS COV-2 EMERGENCE B.1.617 LINEAGES

Coronavirus disease 2019 (COVID-19) is a highly contagious viral disease caused by severe acute respiratory syndrome coronavirus 2 (SARS-CoV-2).[1] As of September 4, 2021, this pandemic has resulted in 4.5 million deaths worldwide, according to the World Health Organization (WHO) (**https://www.who.int/**). Through the efforts of the world's community, the protection of vaccines and effective surveillance of those who have SARS-CoV-2 have significantly reduced the number of COVID-19 hospitalizations as well as deaths. However, in recent months when B.1.617 lineages, especially B.1.617.2 variant (also named Delta) rapidly spread, even though more than five billion vaccine doses have been administered globally (**https://www.who.int/**), thousands of new cases are diagnosed every day. This is why it is essential to have a greater understanding of the SARS CoV-2 Delta variant.

In the case of a typical virus, the rate of its mutation is around 10^{-4} Replacement per site every year. The DNA of the SARS virus appears rather unstable when compared with others RNA viruses. [2] [2]The genetic mutations can cause changes in phenotype that include different antigens, as well as changes in virulence, transmissibility, or. Variants that are more transmissible and resistant to drugs, infectivity, or immune evasion, are more likely to remain during the selection. Thus, a variety of SARS-CoV-2 variants have appeared to replace the existing SARS-CoV-2 variants and have spread across the world. With advantages in competition with their predecessors, these variants are more dominant in many instances. As of now, the current variants have been classified as variants of interest (VOC) or variants of particular

---

1. https://onlinelibrary.wiley.com/doi/full/10.1002/mco2.95#mco295-bib-0001

2.   https://onlinelibrary.wiley.com/doi/full/10.1002/mco2.95#mco295-bib-0002

interest (VOI), according to WHO. VOC contains Alpha (B.1.1.7), Beta (B.1.351), Gamma (P.1), Delta (B.1.617.2) variants (Figure 1 [3]) and their sublineages. VOI includes B.1.525 (Eta), B.1.526 (Iota), B.1.617.1 (Kappa), C.37 (Lambda) and B.1.621 (Mu) variations (**https://www.who.int/en/activities/tracking-SARS-CoV-2-variants**). On August 24, 2021, patients infected with Alpha, Beta, Gamma, and Delta variants were identified across 192, 141 163, and 86 countries, respectively. (**https://apps.who.int/iris/bitstream/handle/10665/344560/CoV-weekly-itrep24Aug21-eng.pdf?sequence=1&isAllowed=y**).

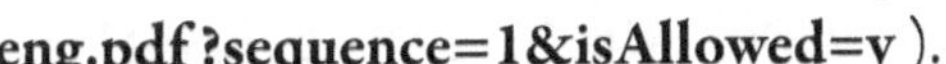

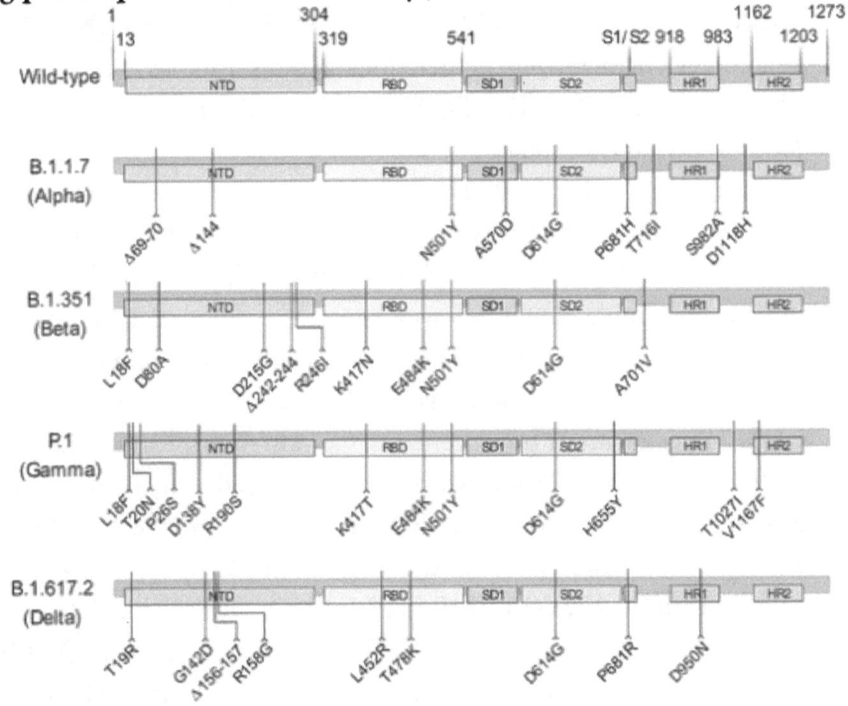

FIGURE 1
Start in the figure viewers PowerPoint

3.   https://onlinelibrary.wiley.com/doi/full/10.1002/mco2.95#mco295-fig-0001

4.   https://onlinelibrary.wiley.com/cms/asset/916c9d52-3ac8-40cd-abac-6bad76c19357/mco295-fig-0001-m.jpg

The diagram shows the changes in spikes in Alpha-beta, Gamma along with Delta variants. Alpha (B.1.1.7) Alpha (B.1.1.7) variation is characterized by deletions at sites 70, 69 as well as 144 within spike. Seven substitutions in spike are N501Y A570D, P681H, D614G T716I, S982A, and D1118H. Beta (B.1.351) variant Beta (B.1.351) variation is characterized by deletions at sites 242-244 and nine substitutions (L18F D80A, L18F, and D215G. R246I are K417N and E484K, as well as N501Y, D614G, as well as the A701V) within spike. Its Gamma (P.1) variation has 12 mutations in spike, and these are L18F, T20N, P26S, and D138Y R190S, K417T E484K, N501Yand D614G H655Y, and T1027I and V1167F. Its Delta (B.1.617.2) variation is characterized by deletions at sites 156, 157, as well as 8 substitutions (T19R G142D, R158G L452R, T478K D614Gand P681R). D950N) in spike

At the beginning of 2021, the variant responsible for the spread of COVID-19 in India was initially referred to as "double mutation" because of E484Q as well as L452R mutations that occurred in spike.4 The name "double mutation" was later changed to B.1.617 because it was several clusters of sequences that shared the common L452R, D614G, and P681R mutations.5 It is important to note that the B.1.617 lineages aren't homogeneous. Certain multiple mutations, like T19R, G142D, or D950N, typically appear together in a lineage. They also are found in other sublineages but at a lesser frequency. Through the sequence of these variants, the first cluster of sequences was found in India with T19R, G142D, L454R E484Q, D614G P681R, as well as D950N mutations in spike.5 The appearance of the Q1071H mutation has led to the formation of B.1.617 lineages, which were split into three subclusters. The first sublineage identified is B.1.617.1 variant (Kappa) and was then B.1.617.2 variation (Delta) as well as B.1.617.3 variant.5 6. B.1.617.1 variant was classified as a VOI by WHO on April 4th, 2021, because of its higher transmission, and the prevalence was reportedly declining. Delta variation was initially identified in October of 2020 in India and then further analysed by March 20, 2021, in the United States. For India, the variant spread quickly, and the percentage of Delta variants in all the sequenced samples increased from 4.0 percent at the time of March 8th, 2021, and 30.4 percent in March 2021, according to the GISAID (**www.gisaid.org**). GISAID WHO identified the Delta variant as a VOI on April 4, 2021. Delta variant as a VOI on the 4th of April 2021. Then, due to its remarkable transmissibility and infectiousness that the Delta variant overtook other previously-existing lineages. Its percentage of all viruses in circulation significantly increased to 89.8 10% on the 10th of May 2021, among the sequences found in India (**www.gisaid.org**). Delta variant was responsible for 17 million COVID-19 cases, which included the recurrence of infections in March and May 2021. 9[5] This result prompted WHO to declare the definition of a VOC as of May 11, 2021. At the moment, B.1.617.3 is neither a VOC nor a VOI due to its low incidence. In essence, B.1.617, along with its sublineages, is responsible for the second cycle of infections that have occurred in India, which resulted in the deaths of more than 30 million COVID-19 patients, and 4000 fatalities from India in the first instance. 10[6]

---

5.   https://onlinelibrary.wiley.com/doi/full/10.1002/mco2.95#mco295-bib-0009

6.   https://onlinelibrary.wiley.com/doi/full/10.1002/mco2.95#mco295-bib-0010

2 COVID-19'S FEATURES INSPIRED by the DELTA VARIANT

The number of receptive cells (R0) of the SARS-CoV-2 wild-type has been calculated to be between 2.3-5.7 (Figure 2A)11 12, 12. Moreover, recent research has revealed that the R0 of the Delta variant can be as high as 8, which is more than Alpha, Beta, and Gamma variants of 55 percent (95 percent CI: 43-68) 60 percent (95% CI: 48-73)) and 34 percent (95 percent of CI 26-43) respectively, 9-13-15 which indicates its high transmission. Delta variant is the most prevalent. Delta variation has taken over existing lineages and is now the most prevalent variation in India and is expected to spread to 163 countries in just a couple of months. While India was fighting COVID-19 infections, a traveller returning from India caused 77% of the sequenced circulating viruses classified as Delta variants in the period between June 2 and 9. in the United Kingdom, where the Alpha variant was first prevalent.7 The benefit of transmission for the Delta variant, as estimated by France, has been found to be 79% more than the Alpha variant.16 At the beginning of August 2021, the percentage of Delta variants in the circulating virus sequences is more than 90% of the world (www.gisaid.org), which causes a new wave of worldwide disease.

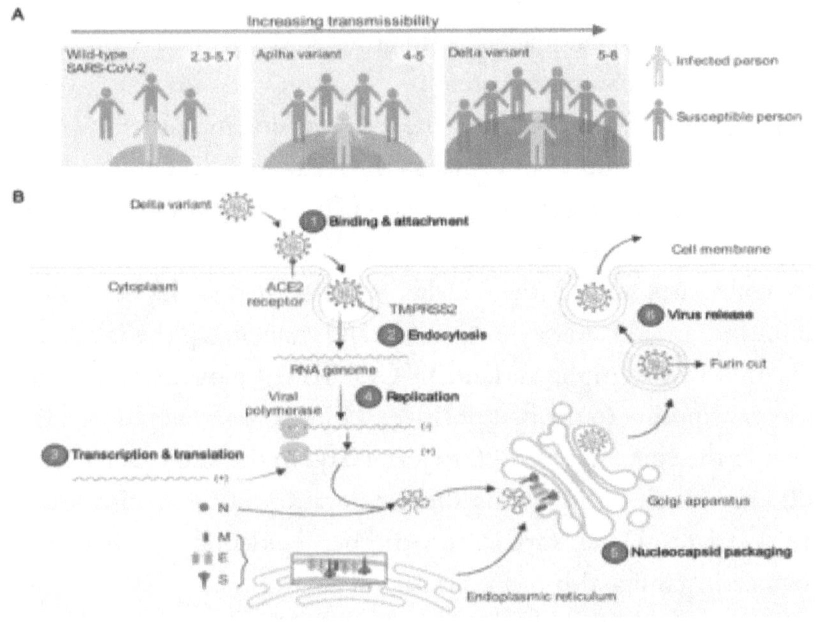

FIGURE 2

Start in the figure viewers PowerPoint

The high transmission and duration of life for Delta variant. Delta variant. (A) Its R0 of the wild-type SARS-CoV-2 virus Alpha variant Delta variants range from 2.3-5.7 5 and 5-8, respectively. (B) Diagrams that are simplified show the process by which the Delta variant gets into and out of cells. A spike in the Delta variant is bound with ACE2 within the host cell. The spike was cut by a transmembrane serine protease (TMPRSS2) to expose components that are required to bind the virus and the host cell membranes. The virus then launches its genome of RNA through the cell of its host, and the viral proteins and RNA are produced. The newly synthesized molecules are processed and packed inside the Golgi apparatus to form the complete virus particle. The spike is then cut by furin, which is an enzyme of the host and allows the virus to attack another cell. A greater proportion of

---

1. https://onlinelibrary.wiley.com/cms/asset/dd2e6dff-cdec-4ad9-8f7d-8d3e5d333e77/mco295-fig-0002-m.jpg

the spike proteins that are variant could be responsible for a higher degree of infection. N: nucleocapsid protein, M: membrane protein, E: envelope protein, S: spike protein

The life-cycle that occurs for the Delta version in cells of the host is illustrated. A mutant variant spike in the Delta variant is more effective in cell entry and increases the development of syncytium. This could result in a higher level of the virus as well as severe illness. Mlcochova and colleagues found that Delta variants had a higher rate of replication in 3D airway organoids and human epithelial airways compared to the Alpha variant. In COVID-19 patients, the interval between exposure to the first positive PCR test has been reduced from 6 days in the epidemic of 2020 to just 4 days in the latest Delta variant outbreak, which indicates the shorter duration of incubation for the Delta variant. Delta variant.18 Another epidemic in Guangdong Province in China also has a similar incubation period.19 The mean generation time and serial intervals are 2.9 as well as 2.3 days respectively, which are less than those of the SARS-CoV-2 wild variant (2.9 as compared to 5.7 to generate a meantime, and 2.3 and 5.5 for the mean serial interval).19 Also, 64.7% (44/68) of the transmission events caused through Delta variants occurred in the presymptomatic period. However, this figure was 59.2 percent in the initial incident in Hubei Province.20 Additionally, The viral burdens of Delta variant infection were, on average, 1000 times higher than those who contracted the infection during the initial outbreak wave.18 In Scotland In Scotland, the Delta variant was observed primarily among younger patients, and the likelihood of hospitalization was roughly twice as high in patients with Delta variant as compared with those suffering from Alpha variant infection.21 In addition, a substantially greater risk of emergency medical hospitalization or attendance was noted within the United Kingdom.16 When taken together, the transmission parameters suggested the likelihood of Delta variant becoming the predominant lineages that circulate and suggest the significant challenges to fight Delta variant.

The features that are characteristic of Delta variation have been examined to determine the reason Delta was able to break through a range of variations. On the one hand, the Delta variant spike fuses more efficiently with target cells with low human angiotensin-converting enzyme 2 (hACE2) levels than other variants, and its pseudovirus infects target cells significantly faster than other variants.22[2] This evolutionary optimization of efficient fusion may explain why the Delta variant can rapidly attack more cells and spread from person to person in a rather short exposure time. However, an analysis of the structure of the RBD's receptor-binding domain reveals that 17 residues of RBD connect with 20 residues in ACE2 to create complex hydrophilic networks that are associated with the virus receptor engagement.23 It is also known that the Delta spike is a shared variant that shares four mutations (L452R, D614G, P681R along with D950N) in common with B.1.617 as well as its sublineage. It also includes five additional mutations (T19R G142D and R158G, D156-D157, and T478K).24 In the present, all circulating variants of SARS-CoV-2 are derived from D614G that plays a role in high susceptibility and infectiousness, however not in terms of disease severity.26-32 L452 residue is located at the edges of the receptor-binding motif (RBM) of RBD. It is directly in connection with ACE2. It is essential for hydrophobicity that it shares with L492 that creates a hydrophobic connection with F490.5 33 L452R modification enhances the infectivity of viruses and fusion efficiency and also the rate of viral replication.34 P681 is found in the distinctive "PRRAR" furin cleavage sites on the S1-S2 boundaries and the S2 boundary. It is a key factor in facilitating the transmission of mutations between humans.23 P681R replacement in the spikes improves the efficiency of the furin cleavage sites and allows for efficient cleavage of

---

2.   https://onlinelibrary.wiley.com/doi/full/10.1002/mco2.95#mco295-bib-0022

the spike through furin, leading to increased syncytium production and increased transmissibility, and pathogenicity.35 36 D950 is located in heptad repetition (HR1) (HR1) of the S2 subunit which is a crucial site which can affect the refolding process of S2. D950 is essential to bind SARS-CoV-2 and the membranes of host cells. 22[3] D950N mutation removes the negative charge that has no apparent effect on the structure of the spike but could increase the fusogenicity of the Delta spike. 22[4] In total, the mutations within the Delta spike are linked to enhance its fitness benefits and pathogenicity as well as the possibility of infection.

3.   https://onlinelibrary.wiley.com/doi/full/10.1002/mco2.95#mco295-bib-0022

4.   https://onlinelibrary.wiley.com/doi/full/10.1002/mco2.95#mco295-bib-0022

3 IMMUNE EVASION OF DELTA VARIANT

The two variations in E484Q and L452R in the sporadic B.1.617 lineages have caused widespread concern since E484 mutations were found in the rapidly expanding varieties Beta as well as Gamma and were linked to immune evasion.5 Studies in the past have revealed that E484 residues were identified as a repulsive molecule in the RBD-ACE2 junction and that mutations in this region could be beneficial to RBD-ACE2 binding.38 Furthermore, E484 and L452 mutations can cause a decline in neutralization by antibodies.39 Thus, B.1.617, B.1.617.1, and B.1.617.3 variants that have E484 as well as L452 mutations were initially thought to be extremely insensitive to the immune system that the human body has. But new research has demonstrated that the vast majority of the serum from convalescents and those who have been vaccinated can block B.1.617 as well as B.1.617.1 variants. The diminution of neutralizing capability is limited to 2 fold. Delta variants were 5.7and 8-fold less sensitive to the serum of vaccinated and convalescent individuals when compared with the wild type.17 41-43 The sera from COVID-19 patients were 4 times less effective against the Delta variant when compared to those of the Alpha variant that was comparable to Beta variants.7 Additionally, the sera of those who had received only one dose of Pfizer or AstraZeneca vaccine showed low neutralizing against the Delta variant. 95% of those who received a complete vaccination had an immune response that neutralized the Delta variant, but the titers of the Delta variant were 3- to 5 times lower than those who had the Alpha variant.7 In a number of clinical studies, the adjusted efficacy (VE) in preventing infection in the people who were fully vaccinated decreased by about 20% for the mRNA vaccine and the adenovirus vector vaccination ChAdOx1.21 The efficacy of the COVID-19 vaccines currently available to fight the Delta variant is summarized in Table 1. In addition, a study conducted recently showed that there was no difference in the viral load between those who were not vaccinated and those who had been fully vaccinated, who may also be infected by the Delta variant. 33% (26/79) of the patients who were infected by the Delta variant displayed a Ct level less than twenty.

TABLE 1. The effectiveness of current COVID-19 vaccines against the Delta variant

Name (company)	Antigen	VE against wild type	Measure outcome	1st Dose VE (95% CI)	2st Dose VE (95% CI)	Country	Reference (Date)
BNT162b2 (Pfizer-BioNTech)	Full-length spike protein with proline substitutions	95%	Symptomatic COVID-19	35.6% (22.7-46.4)	88% (85.3-90.1)	UK	44[1] (21, 20
			Symptomatic infection	56% (45-64)	87% (64-95)	Canada	67[2] (3, 20
			Hospitalization or death	78% (65-86)	—	Canada	
			Hospitalization	94% (46-99)	96% (86-99)	UK	68[3] (14, 20
			Documented infection	30% (17-41)	79% (75-82)	Scotland	21[4] (14, 20
			Symptomatic infection	33.2% (8.3-51.4)	87.9% (78.2-93.2)	UK	58[5] (20, 20
mRNA-1273 (Moderna)	Full-length spike protein with proline substitutions	94.1%	Symptomatic infection	72% (57-82)	—	Canada	67[6] (3, 20
			Hospitalization or death	96% (72-99)	—	Canada	
ChAdOx1 (AZD1222) (AstraZeneca)	Replication-deficient chimpanzee adenoviral vector with the SARS-CoV-2 spike protein	62.1% (two standard doses) 90% (a low dose followed by a standard dose)69[7]	Symptomatic COVID-19	30% (24.3-35.3)	67% (61.3-71.8)	UK	44[8] (21, 20
			Symptomatic infection	67% (44-80)	—	Canada	67[9] (3, 20
			Hospitalization or death	88% (60-96)	—	Canada	
			Hospitalization	71% (51-83)	92% (75-97)	UK	68[10] (4, 20
			Documented	18%	60%	Scotland	21[11]

Name (company)	Antigen	VE against wild type	Measure outcome	1st Dose VE (95% CI)	2st Dose VE (95% CI)	Country	Re
			infection	(9-25)	(53-66)		14
			Symptomatic infection	32.9% (19.3-44.3)	59.8% (28.9-77.3)	UK	58 20

- The data were gathered from WHO as well as PubMed.
- VE, the effectiveness of vaccines; the United Kingdom.

In addition, there is a Delta variant. Delta variant has resistance to certain anti-N-terminal and therapeutic anti-RBD monoclonal antibodies for COVID-19 such as Bamlanivimab. 46[13] However, three other monoclonal antibody Etesivimab, Basirivimab, and Imdevimab, all of which have neutralization capabilities, are still effective to this Delta variant. In addition, using a combination of multiple neutralizing antibodies which recognize and bind to various and nonoverlapping epitopes in the spike might limit the loss of single antibody

1. https://onlinelibrary.wiley.com/doi/full/10.1002/mco2.95#mco295-bib-0044

2. https://onlinelibrary.wiley.com/doi/full/10.1002/mco2.95#mco295-bib-0067

3. https://onlinelibrary.wiley.com/doi/full/10.1002/mco2.95#mco295-bib-0068

4. https://onlinelibrary.wiley.com/doi/full/10.1002/mco2.95#mco295-bib-0021

5. https://onlinelibrary.wiley.com/doi/full/10.1002/mco2.95#mco295-bib-0058

6. https://onlinelibrary.wiley.com/doi/full/10.1002/mco2.95#mco295-bib-0067

7. https://onlinelibrary.wiley.com/doi/full/10.1002/mco2.95#mco295-bib-0069

8. https://onlinelibrary.wiley.com/doi/full/10.1002/mco2.95#mco295-bib-0044

9. https://onlinelibrary.wiley.com/doi/full/10.1002/mco2.95#mco295-bib-0067

10. https://onlinelibrary.wiley.com/doi/full/10.1002/mco2.95#mco295-bib-0068

11. https://onlinelibrary.wiley.com/doi/full/10.1002/mco2.95#mco295-bib-0021

12. https://onlinelibrary.wiley.com/doi/full/10.1002/mco2.95#mco295-bib-0058

13. https://onlinelibrary.wiley.com/doi/full/10.1002/mco2.95#mco295-bib-0046

neutralization and limit the possibility of generating viral escape mutants.47 48

The RBM epitopes of RBD that have a common ACE2 epitope are immunodominant. It is known that T478, E484, and L452 residues are found within immunodominant RBM epitopes that could affect the ability to bind by antibodies from serum or therapeutic antibodies.35 49 L452R modification eliminates the hydrophobic interaction between V105 and I residues in the heavy chain of the antibody, leading to a reduction in neutralization for RBD-specific mAbs.5 Additionally, L452R mutation makes a different epitope peptide structure that reduces the ACE2 and spike and hinders recognition by the T-cell receptors and thus gets rid of the human leukocyte antigen restriction on cell immunity.34 51, T478K mutation is the only one that is unique to the Delta variant. It is located within the epitope region of possible "Class 1" neutralizing monoclonal antibody that binds with the spike protein its closed form. However, the mechanism behind T478K mutation that influences the immune escape process remains unclear. Further research is required to understand the effect it has on. But, these mutations, which include L452R, T478K, and P681R, should be taken into consideration when designing next-generation vaccines or monoclonal antibodies for the future.

4 PERSPECTIVES OF STRATEGIES AGAINST DELTA VARIANT

4.1 Protection from physical damage

WHO has recommended a few measures to safeguard us from COVID-19. This includes washing hands and wearing a face mask, maintaining areas well-ventilated, etc., particularly for healthcare professionals (HCWs) that aren't just working in close proximity to COVID-19 patients but also in an environment that is not well ventilated. Studies have previously revealed that the incidence rates of SARS-CoV-2 among healthcare workers range from 2.2-44 percent, which is substantially greater than that of the general population.53 54, 53 Thus, FFP2/3 and similar respiratory protection devices are suggested to be used in lieu of surgical masks whenever HCWs interact with COVID-19 patients to minimize the risk of secondary transmission of the virus, especially when dealing with high-infectious variants such as Delta.54-56 Additionally, those who have occupational exposure to SARS-CoV-2 must be encouraged to perform frequent tests to reduce the risk of spread.

4.2 Optimizing vaccination program

Research has shown that an existing cellular immune system in individuals who are infected with other coronaviruses could cause a difference in the degree of disease in COVID-19 patients, 57[1] that could explain why those who have fully vaccinated exhibit moderately milder phenotypes for COVID-19 when compared with those who have not been vaccinated. Similar to this, though a decrease in VE for the Delta variant was found in several studies, vaccines currently available are still effective against the Delta variant.58 For instance, those who had have received at least one dose of vaccine were 50percent less likely to contract SARS-CoV-2 than nonvaccinated members.59

---

1. https://onlinelibrary.wiley.com/doi/full/10.1002/mco2.95#mco295-bib-0057

In the case of COVID-19 cases that were associated with outbreaks in central Oklahoma, the majority (40/47) did not receive any dose of COVID-19 vaccination; however, 6percent (3/47) or 9 percent (4/47) had received a single dose, and 2 doses Moderna or Pfizer BioNTech vaccines.15 These results suggest that vaccination is a reliable method to prevent Delta variant infections. The development of vaccines based upon the Delta spike could significantly improve the efficacy of vaccines in protecting against. Prior to the use of the Delta-specific vaccine, optimizing our vaccination regimen could be a viable strategy to boost the effectiveness of the VE for the Delta variant. Combining a DNA-based vaccine as well as a recombinant subunit vaccine resulted in an increase in nAbs levels and robust T-cell immune responses that protect macaques in rhesus after the attack of SARS-CoV-2 viruses that is superior to the administration of protein vaccine or DNA on their own. 60[2] and Georg Behrens, an immunologist at the Hanover Medical School in Germany He pointed out that vaccination using different types of vaccines can result in a more robust overall response, which could increase the efficacy.

Additionally, nasal and oral mucosae function as the primary defense against pathogens that prevent their entering and infection.62 The research and the lessons from MERS-CoV and SARS-CoV suggest that activation of mucosal immune responses is an effective method to reduce the severity of SARS-CoV-2, particularly in the case of the Delta variant, which has less resistance to vaccines as compared to the Beta variant but exhibits a high transmission and infectivity.63-65 Thus, the development of COVID-19 vaccines that trigger an immune response that is strong to both mucosal sites as well as the systemic circulation could be a feasible strategy to reduce the severity of infection and transmission of the Delta variant.

---

2.   https://onlinelibrary.wiley.com/doi/full/10.1002/mco2.95#mco295-bib-0060

Infections and Spread

The Delta variant is more prone to infection and is more prevalent than earlier variants of SARS-CoV-2, a virus that causes COVID-19.

- **This Delta variation is far more infectious:** The Delta variant is extremely contagious, with more than two times as contagious as the previous variants.

- **A few studies suggest that the Delta variant could cause more severe illnesses than other variants that have been seen in non-vaccinated individuals.** In two different studies conducted in Canada and Scotland, patients who were infected by this Delta variant are more likely to require hospitalization as compared to those infected with Alpha or the virus which causes COVID-19. Yet the vast majority of deaths and hospitalizations caused by COVID-19 are for those who have not been vaccinated.

- **People who are not vaccinated are the biggest risk to consider:** The greatest risk of transmission occurs among non-vaccinated individuals who are more likely to contract the virus and thus transmit the virus. People who have fully vaccinated contract COVID-19 (known as breakthrough infections) much less often than those who are not vaccinated. Patients infected by Delta variants of COVID Delta variant, such as those who have been fully vaccinated and suffer from an asymptomatic breakout infection, are able to pass the infection on to other people. CDC continues to analyze information on whether fully-vaccinated patients suffering from asymptomatic breakthrough diseases are able to carry the disease.

- Completely vaccinated individuals who suffer from Delta variant breakthroughs can transmit the virus to others. However, those who are vaccinated appear to be able to spread the virus less frequently. In the case of prior variants, smaller amounts of genetic material were detected in the blood samples of those who were fully vaccinated and had breakthrough infections than those from COVID-19 sufferers. For those who are infected with COVID-19, the Delta variant, the same quantities of genetic material from the virus were found in both nonvaccinated and fully vaccinated individuals. But, as with other variants, the quantity of genetic material from the virus could be reduced more quickly in fully vaccinated individuals as compared to people who have not been vaccinated. So, people who have been fully vaccinated will likely contract the virus in a shorter period of time than those who are not vaccinated.

Vaccines

Vaccines used in the US are extremely effective and include the Delta variant

- The COVID-19 vaccinations that are approved or approved by the United States are highly effective at preventing severe illness and death, which includes that Delta variant. However, they're not 100% effective, and some who are fully vaccinated are susceptible to becoming infected (called "breakthrough" infection) and developing an illness. In all cases who are vaccinated, it is the most effective protection against disease and death.

- Vaccines play a vital role in preventing the spreading of this virus and in reducing serious illness. Although they are highly efficient, they aren't 100% effective, and there could be breakthrough vaccine-related infections. Millions of Americans are vaccinated, and the numbers are growing. This means that, even though the risk of developing breakthrough infections is minimal, there will be many fully vaccinated individuals who contract the disease and are able to spread the disease to others, especially because of the increased spreading of the Delta variant. In certain communities has led to the rapid increase in cases of this Delta variant, and this increases the likelihood that more dangerous variants may emerge.

- Immunization is the best option to safeguard yourself, your family members, and the community. The high rate of vaccination can reduce transmission of the disease as well as prevent the emergence of new variants. CDC suggests that all people 12 years or older be vaccinated as soon as is possible.

While many began to have a glimmer of hope—or at least cautious optimism, early this summer, that the virus could be fading into the background, there was the risk that new mutations in the COVID-19 virus could trigger it again and make it more potent.

Then then, the Delta variant was discovered in The United States. The first time it was discovered in India in the latter half of the year 2020, Delta quickly spread across the country as well as Great Britain before reaching the U.S., where it rapidly grew. The virus was, up until mid-December, the most prevalent SARS CoV-2 variant, accounting for more than 90% instances of COVID-19 (at the time of the) and causing an unprecedented increase in hospitalizations across a number of states. (Omicron is currently the most common version within America. The U.S.)

Delta is thought to be more than two times more contagious than prior variants. Additionally, studies have proven that it might become a more likely original virus to place patients in the hospital. People who have not been vaccinated are the most susceptible, and the greatest incidence of cases and the most severe consequences are seen in regions where there are low vaccination rates.

Inci Yildirim, MD Ph.D. who is the Yale Medicine Paediatric Infectious Diseases Specialist and vaccinologist, didn't feel shocked by the progression of Delta's disease. "All viruses evolve over time and undergo changes as they spread and replicate," she says.

As of this time, those who have been fully vaccine-vaccinated against coronavirus continue to be protected against COVID-19 as compared to people who aren't. However, there are plenty of questions that cause the Centres for Disease Control and Prevention (CDC) to suggest additional precautions. This includes mask guidelines, regardless of vaccination status, and recommendations regarding the booster shot.

Although the majority of Delta cases have occurred among those who haven't been vaccinated, research also has shown the Delta variant to be more susceptible to transmission even among those who have been vaccinated.

Based on the CDC that if a person is infected by COVID-19 (in what's known as "breakthrough" or "breakthrough" case) and suffers from symptoms, they may transmit the virus to other people. The agency is looking into the data regarding whether people who are fully vaccinated can transmit the virus even when they are in an outbreak but have no signs.

Here are five things that you should be aware of about the Delta version.

1. Delta is more infectious than other strains of the virus.

The CDC has classified Delta **"a variant of concern[1],"** making use of the same designation for the Alpha strain, which first surfaced on the scene in Great Britain, the Beta strain first surfacing within South Africa, and the Gamma strain discovered in Brazil. (The new name conventions for variants were developed in the World Health Organization [WHO] as an alternative to the numerical names.)

The rapid growth rate of Delta has been particularly impressive, according to F. Perry Wilson, MD, an Yale Medicine epidemiologist. Delta was spread 50% more quickly than Alpha and was 50% more infectious than the SARS-CoV-2 original strain, the doctor says. "In a completely unmitigated environment—where no one is vaccinated or wearing masks—it's estimated that the average person infected with the original coronavirus strain will infect 2.5 other people," Dr Wilson says. "In the same environment, Delta would spread from one person to maybe 3.5 or 4 other people."

"Because of the math, it grows exponentially and more quickly," the doctor declares. "So, what seems like a fairly modest rate of infectivity can cause a virus to dominate very quickly."

2. People who have not been vaccinated are at risk.

Within the U.S., there is a disproportionate amount of unvaccinated citizens within Southern as well as Appalachian states, including Alabama, Arkansas, Georgia, Mississippi, Missouri, and

---

1.   https://www.cdc.gov/coronavirus/2019-ncov/variants/variant-info.html#Concern

West Virginia, where vaccination rates are not high; however, the number of cases is rising across the country too. The month of September saw health professionals in Idaho have one of the lowest rates of vaccination across the country, increased restrictions on health care throughout the state following the Delta outbreak caused the shortage of health care resources for all patients in hospitals.

Teenagers, children as well as young adults pose a threat as well. "A study from the United Kingdom showed that children and adults under 50 were 2.5 times more likely to become infected with Delta," the doctor Dr. Yildirim. It is known that the U.S. has allowed Pfizer-BioNTech vaccinations for adolescents and teens since May. Then, at the beginning of November, the CDC approved FDA authorization for Pfizer's Pfizer vaccine to children aged 5-17.

"As older age groups get vaccinated, those who are younger and unvaccinated will be at higher risk of getting COVID-19 with **any variant**[2]," says Dr. Yildirim. "But Delta seems to be impacting younger age groups more than previous variants."

3. Delta and Omicron could cause hyperlocal outbreaks.'

If Omicron, Delta, and Omicron continue to speed up the spread of the disease, the doctor. Wilson says the biggest concerns will be related to the higher risk of transmission. The answer will depend, in part, the location you reside in and the number of people living in your area who are vaccinated, he adds. "I call it 'patchwork vaccination,' where you have these pockets that are highly vaccinated that are adjacent to places that have 20% vaccination," Dr Wilson says. "The problem is that this allows the virus to hop, skip, and jump from one poorly vaccinated area to another."

In certain instances, towns that are not vaccinated and are located in high-vaccination regions could be hit with the virus within its boundaries, and the outcome could result in "hyperlocal outbreaks," he

---

2.   https://www.yalemedicine.org/news/coronavirus-variants

declares. "Then, the pandemic could look different than what we've seen before, where there are real hotspots around the country."

Therefore, instead of a three or four-year epidemic that dies out after a certain number of people have been vaccination-free, the increase in cases could be compressed to a shorter period. "That sounds almost like a *good* thing," Dr Wilson says. "It's not." If more people get sick all at once in one region, the health care system could become overwhelmed, and more patients are likely to die, he states. "That's something we have to worry about a lot."

4. There's still a lot to discover about Delta.

As the information on Delta is accumulating, researchers are striving to understand the most information possible in the shortest time possible. A key question is whether Delta is a Delta strain that can cause you to be sicker as the primary virus. The first information on the degree that came from Delta included studies of Scotland in Scotland and Canada that were both referenced by the CDC and suggested that the Delta variant is more likely to cause hospitalization among those who have not been vaccinated. A study in the summer of 2009 was that was published in *The Lancet Infectious Diseases*[3] discovered that those who resided in England who had Delta were twice as likely to be hospitalized chance of those with Alpha which was the predominant mutation in the country.

Another concern is the way Delta impacts the body. There are reports of symptoms distinct from those that are associated with the coronavirus strain that was originally identified, Dr Yildirim states. "It seems like cough and loss of smell are less common," she declares. "And headache, sore throat, runny nose, and fever are presently based on surveys in the U.K."

In the meantime, experts continue to investigate Delta in addition to the cases that are breakthrough. It's not easy to pinpoint the exact

---

3.   *https://www.thelancet.com/journals/laninf/article/PIIS1473-3099(21)00475-8/*

fulltext

numbers of these illnesses across the U.S., where the CDC has stopped not counting cases that do not result in death or hospitalization in May. The agency says that no vaccine is 100 percent effective. Any increase in cases could have an associated increase in cases of breakthrough infections.

There are other concerns and questions about Delta and Delta Plus, which includes **Delta Plus**[4]—a subvariant of Delta which is found throughout countries like the U.S., the U.K., and in other nations. "Delta Plus has one additional mutation to what the Delta variant has," Dr. Yildirim says. Dr. Yildirim. The mutation, known as K417N, is a problem with the spike protein which the virus requires to spread its virus to cells and is the primary goal of the mRNA as well as various vaccines, she adds.

"Delta Plus has been reported initially in India However, the form of mutation was identified in other variants like Beta, which first emerged. More research is required to determine the true extent of the spread and the impact of this variant on the burden of disease and outcomes," Dr Yildirim continues.

5. Vaccination is your best defense against Delta.

The most important thing you can do to protect yourself from Delta is to get fully vaccinated, the doctors say. The CDC endorses a clinical preference for a vaccination with the Pfizer and Moderna shots, both of which are two-dose vaccines. You must get both of those shots and then wait the recommended two-week period for them to take full effect. All adults are eligible to be vaccinated (as well as children as young as 5 for the Pfizer-BioNTech vaccine). Boosters are also recommended.

Even though fully vaccinated individuals who have a breakthrough illness are able to spread the virus to others and spread the virus to others, the CDC says they have a lower amount of virus genetic material that could decrease more quickly in people who are

---

4.   https://www.yalemedicine.org/news/dont-call-it-delta-plus

vaccinated. As a result, although they've been shown to have similar amounts of viruses in their throats and noses as those who have not been vaccinated, research has also revealed that they could transmit the virus for less period of time.

There are other CDC prevention guidelines that are available to both vaccinations as well as non-vaccinated individuals. In the process of vaccinating more people across this part of the U.S., the CDC recommends "layered prevention strategies" for everyone, and this includes wearing masks for the face when in public indoor environments in areas of significant and high risk of transmission. The agency has also suggested universal indoor masking to all staff, students, teachers, and students visiting K-12 schools. There could also be mandates for masks in accordance with your location.

"Like everything in life, this is an ongoing risk assessment," said Dr Yildirim. "If it's hot and you'll be out in the sun, then you should put on some sunscreen. If you're in a crowd and you are likely to be with non-vaccinated persons, then you put your mask on and maintain your social from interacting. If you're unvaccinated and not eligible to receive this vaccine, "the most effective option is to be vaccine-free."

Of course, there are a lot of individuals who have not received the vaccine due to personal circumstances or issues that have caused obstacles, or they decide not to take the vaccine. What do you think? Will the Delta version suffice to convince those who are able to be vaccinated? There's no way to know for certain; however, it is possible, claims Dr Wilson, who encourages anyone who is unsure about vaccination to consult their doctor of choice.

"When there are local outbreaks, vaccine rates go up," Dr Wilson says. "We know that if a person you know becomes seriously sick and is admitted into the hospital for treatment, that might alter the risk assessment slightly. It could happen more frequently. I'm hopeful we see vaccine rates go up."

Omicron Variant:

Between the 26th of November and 12th December 2021 (17:00) Between 26 November and 12 December 2021 at 17:00, 5 435 verified Omicron VOC cases were reported across 69 countries around the world, from publicly available data (including the ones that were reported in the form of GISAID). Of these cases

23 EU/EEA nations have reported 766 cases on the basis of the results of sequencing: Austria (17), Belgium (30), Croatia (3),

Cyprus (3), Czechia (5), Denmark (195), Estonia (15), Finland (20), France (59), Germany (82), Greece (3),

Iceland (20), Ireland (6), Italy (13), Latvia (5), Liechtenstein (1), the Netherlands (62), Norway (109), Portugal

(49), Romania (7), Slovakia (3), Spain (36), and Sweden (23), according to public sources. Additionally, Denmark and Germany have reported 1 36 and 645 cases, respectively which were confirmed with a PCR that is specific to the variant. Numerous cases that could be related to the variant have been reported across several countries.

While the majority of reported cases were first related to travel, an increasing proportion of cases are being reported as coming from the EU/EEA area and as part of clusters or outbreaks. Some cases are being discovered by representative sampling in regular surveillance systems. For all cases that have data on the severity of the illness were classified as mild or non-symptomatic. There have not been any Omicron-related deaths yet reported within the European Union/Eurasian Economic Area. However, these numbers should be viewed with caution since the numbers of cases confirmed are low, and it's still too early to determine the emergence of severe diseases in a large number of recently discovered cases to know whether the spectrum of clinical manifestations for Omicron differs from the previously identified variants. The countries in the EU/EEA reporting cases that do not have any epidemiological connection to travel outside of the EU/EEA region include Belgium and Denmark, France (TESSy), Finland, Spain, Iceland, and Sweden. This suggests that the transmission of community-wide is ongoing in the EU/EEA Members States. Between November 26 and December 2021, various clusters and outbreaks have been identified by at least 11 EU/EEA nations, including Belgium; the other countries are Belgium, Cyprus, Croatia, Denmark, Finland, France, Iceland, Ireland, Italy, Norway, Portugal Romania, and Spain. The clusters are linked to family gatherings as well as business gatherings, sports teams conferences, Christmas celebrations, and other gatherings. The size of clusters varied from two or 123 instances, with confirmed cases and possible cases. In a massive outbreak discovered in Norway, it was reported that the majority of participants received two doses of the vaccine. There was also evidence that cases have received vaccinations in other groups (e.g., Romania).

States and territories that are not part of the EU/EEA region have reported confirmed cases of Omicron. These 43 territories that have reported confirmed cases include Argentina, Australia, Bangladesh, Botswana, Brazil, Canada, Chile, Cuba, Hong Kong Special Administrative Region, Fiji, Ghana, India, Israel, Japan, Jordan, Kuwait, Lebanon, Malawi,

Malaysia, Maldives, Mexico, Namibia, Nepal, Nigeria, Russia, Saudi Arabia, Senegal, Sierra Leone, Singapore, South

Africa, South Korea, Sri Lanka, Switzerland, Taiwan, Thailand, Tunisia, Turkey, Uganda, United Arab Emirates,

United Kingdom (including cases reported in Bermuda and Gibraltar), United States of America, Zambia, and Zimbabwe. In the WHO European Region, one death that was confirmed as having Omicron VOC was reported in the UK, according to an article in the media that quoted authorities on the 13th of December, 2021. The same media report included around 10 hospitalizations involving Omicron VOC.

Molecular properties

Omicron VOC Omicron VOC belongs to the Pango lineage B.1.1.529 It is distinguished through 21 amino acid modifications of the spike protein as compared with the virus that was originally discovered (G142D G339D, G339D. S373P K417N. N440K. S477N, T478Kand E484A Q493R, Q498R N501Y, Y505Hand D614G H655Y. N679K. P681H. N764K. D796Y, and Q954H. N969K). Of these modifications, 12 of them are found in the receptor-binding region (RBD) (residues 319-541).

The lineage B.1.1.529 is currently divided into 2 sub-lineages: BA.1 (B.1.1.529.1) as well as BA.2 (B.1.1.529.2) 2929. Alongside the distinctive mutation that is found in B.1.1.529, BA.1 is characterized by other differences with respect to the spike protein (A67V D69-70 T95I), D143-145, N211I, D212, and ins215EPE, G446S, S371L, G496S

T547K. N856K. L981F.) and BA.2 are distinguished by a different set of distinctions (T19I L24S, D25-27 V213G. S371F. T376A, R408S, D405N). It is important to note that BA.2 does not contain D69-70 protein in the spike protein, which is why it is not detected by the S-gene target Failure (SGTF) as measured by the Thermo Fischer TaqPath test. As of December 12, 2021, The BA.1 lineage is home to the vast majority of B.1.1.529 sequences (1545/1452, 99.5%) accessible from GISAID EpiCoV. All evidence that supports the phenotypical characteristics of Omicron currently available originates directly from the BA.1 lineage and is not entirely relevant in BA.2 lineage. BA.2 lineage.

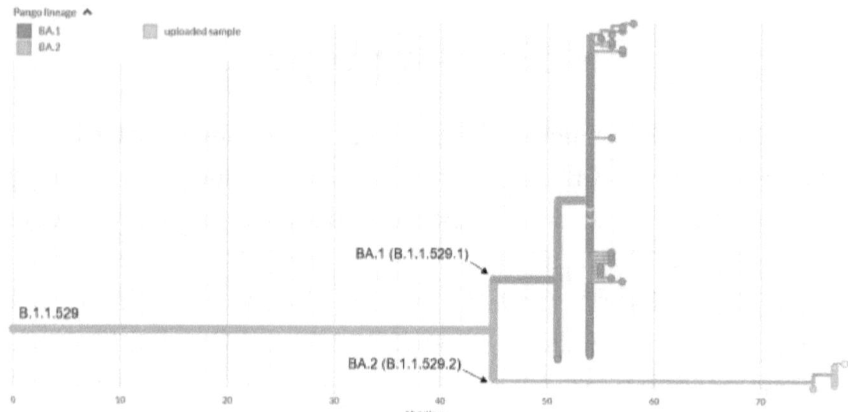

The tree was created by using an UShER internet interface (http://30.30.30.30.30.30.30.30. EPI_ISL_7259716 was the query sequence. One hundred samples were chosen by the tool to illustrate the position of the query in relation to the entire SARS-CoV-2 tree.

Transmissibility

Omicron VOC Omicron VOC displays a significant improvement in its growth rate in comparison to Delta VOC. Delta VOC and is likely to beat that of the Delta VOC (see section 'Forecasts for Omicron VOC epidemiology'). According to UK information that Omicron VOC has a higher risk of secondary attack, Omicron VOC has an increased risk of transmission to the household, a higher secondary attack rate, and a higher growth rate in comparison with Delta (31). Based on these results, an adjusted risk ratio of household transmissions of one Omicron VOC index case, compared to a Delta VOC index case, from routine testing results, was found as 3.2 (95 percent 95% confidence interval 2.0-5.0). The odds ratio (OR) for close contacts becoming secondary was 2.09 (95 percent 95% CI 1.54-2.79). The rate of secondary attacks in the household for secondary attacks in the UK was calculated to be 21.6 percent (95 percent range of 16.7-27.4%)) in Omicron VOC. Omicron VOC, compared to 10.7 percent (95 percent range of 10.5-10.8 percent) of the Delta VOC. There were, however, several limitations to these studies, such as the insufficient adjustment for vaccination, the status of contacts' prior infections, and the possibility of bias in ascertainment. Thus, the initial results must be taken with caution.

The data collected from South Africa continue to confirm Omicron's advantage in growth over other variations. Cases confirmed to continue to increase in affected areas within South Africa, and in the Gauteng province, rates of cases are increasing more quickly than the previous waves. Between mid-August, too late October 2021, the effective reproduction number (Rt) within South Africa was estimated at less than 1. Then, it increased dramatically up to 2.2 (95 percent CI 1.96-2.43) in mid-November, accompanied by an increase in new diagnoses. As the number of cases increased, an increase in the percentage of samples that had S-gene deletion was observed as a determinant indicator of the presence of Omicron VOC. Omicron VOC. The percentage then increased dramatically from 10% to95 percentage in the month of November 2021.

In the UK In the UK, the percentage of cases that have SGTF (now extremely predictive of Omicron) continues to increase quickly. The growth rate estimated for Omicron's VOC based upon adjusted SGTF counts was, as of December 2021, at 35 percent per day. In the week prior to week 47 number of cases containing SGTF throughout the UK had been typically under 150, which made less than 0.1 percent of all cases. In the case of week 48 that was dated from the 30th of November, 2021, and onwards, the total number of cases that had SGTF that were in the UK has already risen to 705 (31). Based on the current increase rate of 5%, the UK has predicted that Omicron VOC case numbers will be comparable to Delta VOC cases by mid-December in the UK. In different studies and research, the initial process of doubling of South Africa was estimated as 1 to 2 days, and the doubling period in Denmark at the time of 9 December 20, 2021, was estimated to be between 2-4 days. This is comparable to the estimates by the UK.

These studies show it is true that the Omicron VOC has a growth advantage when compared with other variants, like those of the Delta VOC. But there are uncertainties in the present estimates of transmissibility. Further studies are required to provide accurate estimates of the transmission of the entire variant and also in relation to measures that are in place in various environments of the community.

Severity

There is not enough data available to assess at present with certainty the severity of the disease that is caused by Omicron VOC in comparison to other common variants. However, until now, serious cases have been relatively rare across the EU/EEA. In the first Omicron VOC cases reported by the close of week 48-2021, EU/EEA nations to TESSy 70 percent (122/174) were symptoms. From those more than 117 Omicron VOC cases for which hospitalization data was reported, there was only one classified as being hospitalized, and no instances were reported as admitted to an ICU or dying. The majority of EU/EEA patients were discovered in the last few days and, if symptoms were present, they had very recent signs of onset. Additionally, the majority of cases with a date of birth available were young. 74 percent (128/174) comprised between the ages of 20-49 years old. age. Since at least a part of the cases involved traveller-related or associated with outbreaks in the context of social interaction, they could also be believed to be healthy when compared to the general population. Information on the status of vaccination was inaccessible for the vast majority of the cases.

The data obtained from Gauteng province in South Africa indicate a rise in hospital admissions for COVID-19 patients, ranging from

In week 45, there were 153 cases to 2201 cases in week 48. Then there were deaths between 18 deaths during week 45 up to 83 death during week 49. The increase is associated with the growing prevalence of the Omicron variant in the COVID-19 cases reported. Although the rate of cases is increasing more rapidly than in prior waves within the Gauteng province, the hospitalization rate is increasing as well, in line with previous waves. This suggests that the rise in hospital admissions is the result of the higher number of cases instead of being due to an increase in severity. Based on an analysis of 211 000 positive COVID-19 cases in the Omicron outbreak, adults have less of a risk-adjusted for vaccination status in comparison to the initial wave of infection that was dominated by D614G in the year 2020. The high levels of seropositivity within South Africa prior to the Omicron VOC wave could potentially cause a lower severity of the disease in this population, even though cases-linked information on prior infection or vaccinations aren't available.

In a case of infection linked to a Christmas celebration in Norway, 80 out of 111 guests were identified with SARS-CoV2. Of the 80 people (mostly between 30 to 50 years of age) who were fully vaccinated and classified as likely SARSCoV 2 Omicron Cases of the VOC) All but one were diagnosed with symptoms. The majority of these 79 patients reported coughing or headache, fatigue, and sore throat. Nearly half of them reported fever. The time of onset for symptoms was usually three days following the event. There have been no hospital admissions to the date been recorded. It is nevertheless crucial to remember that serious results can take weeks to build up and take longer to become evident at a population level, affecting the rate of hospitalization. The current estimates of Omicron VOC severity are still undetermined, and further studies that include a longer-term follow-up by age, prior infections, and the vaccination status of those who have been discovered are required to give more accurate estimates.

Potential for immune escape

Omicron is one of the more genetically distinct SARS-CoV-2 types that has been detected in significant amounts in the current pandemic. It has been a source of concern that it could be linked with a significant decrease in the efficacy of vaccines and monoclonal antibodies, in addition to the risk of SARS-CoV-2 infections that recur. Numerous changes in the sequence that codes for the spike protein have already been reported and are linked to an escape of the immune response from neutralizing antibodies, The sequence of the spike protein is known to be associated with an immune escape from neutralizing antibodies.

The pre-prints, which are peer-reviewed but not peer-reviewed, available suggest that the neutralization capabilities of the vaccinee (primary course) and convalescent sera against Omicron are significantly diminished compared to the previous SARS-CoV-2 VOC. There is evidence to suggest that the neutralization of virus through sera of individuals who have had the combination of infection and complete vaccine (primary course) or those with booster shots are at most partially effective for the neutralization of Omicron in vitro. These early neutralization results suggest that there is a reduction in the effectiveness of vaccines, especially regarding how it prevents infection. However, these findings must be confirmed using larger samples and additional laboratories for patients who have diverse clinical characteristics (brand of the vaccine, other doses of vaccine, the intensity of the infection) as well as sampling times after an infection or vaccination.

It is challenging to directly convert in vitro neutralization findings into clinical outcomes, such as protection against infection or severe disease, in which case robust effectiveness of vaccines and breakthrough infection information are essential in clinical environments. There is no definitive threshold of antibody titer that has been identified as a measure of SARS-CoV-2 protection. The lower neutralizing antibody titers in serum samples taken within three to six months following vaccination or infection may be compensated for by the persistence of virus-specific, long-lived T cells, which are able to quickly expand following subsequent infections to produce higher neutralizing antibody amounts and, In addition, the role of the conserved non-neutralizing antibody and memory T-cell responses has not been assessed by in vitro neutralization studies, yet it is possible that they aid in protecting from a severe illness in the case of severe disease.

Therapeutics

Presently, only limited information is available on monoclonal antibodies to treat Omicron. Pre-print information that is not peer-reviewed shows that the mixture of casirivimab with imdevimab fails to neutralize Omicron in the laboratory, while the ability of sotrovimab to neutralize remains against Omicron. The initial genetic analysis of antiviral remdesivir suggests that it could remain active against Omicron, but this has not yet been confirmed by tests in the laboratory. The clinical and laboratory evidence on the efficacy of more recent antiviral medications for oral use against Omicron is not yet available.

Testing in the laboratory

While RT-PCR tests continue to be the gold standard for COVID-19 testing due to their high specificity and sensitivity, many EU/EEA nations have begun a RADT test as well as self-RADTs to increase their testing capabilities overall. Despite the rise of viruses with variants, however, no decline in the sensitivity of tests using RADTs has been documented in the past (57). **Preliminary results of the fast assessment conducted by the Foundation for Innovative New Diagnostics (FIND) suggest their sensitivity used for diagnosis of infection hasn't been affected by the development from the Omicron version.** In addition, the first laboratory-based evaluation for lateral flow machines used in use by the NHS in the UK's NHS (National Health Service) Test and Trace has found similar sensitivity when it comes to finding Omicron similar to Delta. It is crucial to remember that further studies of the performance of RADTs that detect Omicron have not yet been conducted. Omicron variants in environments that have high transmission levels have not yet been completed. More studies are in progress, and laboratories must be vigilant to look for decreases in the sensitiveness of RADTs that are used to identify different VOCs. More information about the use of RADTs may be read in the revised ECDC Technical Report.

RT-PCR-based S-gene Target Failure (SGTF) tests that do not detect the S-gene that carries an insertional deletion D6970 could be utilized to test for VOCs in the Omicron VOC. However, it must be pointed out that a recently identified Omicron sublineage BA.2 (B.1.1.529.2) is described, which does not carry the mutation D69-70. Even though only a tiny amount of BA.2 sequences have been discovered in the world, care is recommended in using SGTF tests since viruses from this sub-lineage won't be detected using these tests. It is worth noting that there are very few sequences of non-Omicron lineage virus which contain D69-70. So, a small portion of

SGTF-screened cases must be considered for further confirmation sequencing.

Screening for specific amino acid substitutions can be performed by using specific RT-PCR tests that target SNPs; It is also possible to screen for specific amino acid substitutions. **However, it is imperative to keep in mind that current SNP tests might not detect or identify newly emerging variants carrying the particular SNP because of amino acid substitutions at neighboring sites which affect the binding of the probe and primer.** In the case of the Omicron variant, in particular, it has been observed that commercially-available SNP tests for the detection of T478K P681H, N501Y, and T478K cannot reliably detect the mutations, despite the possibility that the variant has mutations in the S gene. The US FDA has released the following list of molecular tests which could be affected by SARS-CoV-2 mutations Omicron variant. Similar to this, the Joint Research Centre (JRC) monitors the effectiveness of RT-PCR test assays and provides data in the JRC Dashboard (61). Analyses of in silico carried out by JRC have revealed six assays that are not able to detect or are less sensitive up to Omicron (62). Laboratory personnel is encouraged to test the efficacy of protocols utilized on dashboards that deal with in silico analysis as well as clinical validations.

Other assays have been created to identify the presence of Omicron (e.g., that focuses on S371L/S373P).

(Ins214EPE and E484A) (63, 64E484A and ins214EPE). A complete listing of methods for identifying the Omicron variant, as well as an accompanying table of amino acids that are substituted, deleted, or inserted to facilitate the analysis of various VOCs, are available within Annexes 1 2 and 1, respectively. WHO is the WHO's Regional Office for Europe, and ECDC has created an information-sharing protocol, EZCollab, to facilitate 'COVID-19 protocol sharing' between national public health labs. Registration can be made at: https://ezcollab.who.int/euroflu/flulab/covid19_protocols.[1]

---

1. https://ezcollab.who.int/euroflu/flulab/covid19_protocols

Public perceptions

There is currently no information about public opinions about Omicron specifically. This means that we don't yet know how this new variant could impact people's desire to adhere to current NPIs or their acceptance or uptake of the COVID-19 vaccine. More data collection is required to gain a better understanding of whether the perceptions people have of Omicron can inspire them to take on greater personal protection or even to be vaccinated. Although not specifically related to Omicron, the data collected from Belgium between the end of November and the beginning of December indicated an increase in awareness of a 'high risk of infection in the population studied. Researchers speculated that this rise could be due to increased awareness of the current health situation that included the disclosure of Omicron cases across Europe. In addition, the WHO-EARS social listening tool detected an uptick in a number of topics COVID-19 variants more than any other topic in the last 30 days. In addition, in response to concerns identified by social listening, researchers at the Robert Koch Institute have updated its COVID-19 FAQs, which include the potential impact Omicron might influence the effectiveness of vaccines. In summation, even though the public's understanding of and perception of the potential risks posed by Omicron remains to be thoroughly mapped, however, there are signs of concern regarding the current situation about the COVID-19 epidemic.

Vaccines (effectiveness declining evidence to support boosters)

The mutations found on the Omicron VOC specifically within the binding area in the spike protein indicate a potential for the escape of vaccines by this variant, compared to that of the Delta VOC. As mentioned above, the preliminary in vitro research suggests a diminished neutralization capability for Omicron VOC. Omicron VOC, although large uncertainties remain. However, the protection conferred by COVID-19 vaccinations doesn't only rely on antibodies to the RBD in the spike protein of SARS-CoV-2. Immunity induced by vaccines directed to epitopes that are not part of the RBD could play a significant role in preventing severe disease after infection with Omicron.

In terms of protection from vaccines against transmission onward, infection and infections with milder disease the fact that is neutralizing antibodies are greatly altered by the Omicron VOC indicates that prior infections or vaccination could have reduced protection against these outcomes in particular if antibody levels decrease in time. More studies of the clinical efficacy of boosters against Omicron VOC are urgently required (to this point, only one study has been published) and more research and actual data regarding Omicron VOC's effect. Omicron VOC on waning immunity after vaccination or natural infection. This is the only way to make it possible to comprehend Omicron's impact on the effectiveness of vaccines fully.

Actual data on the efficacy of the vaccines approved by the EU against Omicron VOC are not yet available except for some preliminary estimates regarding the possibility of vaccine efficacy against symptoms of disease caused by the Omicron VOC. Moderate-to-high effectiveness of the vaccine against COVID-19-related symptoms is described in the first few days after administering a booster dose with Comirnaty (70-75 percent). These findings strongly support using a dose booster in conjunction with the full course of the vaccination program as a method to protect against symptomatic illness due to the Omicron VOC. As noted by the authors, the study, which is yet to be peer-reviewed, was conducted at an extremely infancy stage before the appearance of Omicron and had a range of drawbacks. This highlights the significance and necessity of more studies of the effectiveness of vaccines on larger numbers of people.

There have been reports of SARS-CoV-2 reinfections that involve Omicron VOC. Omicron VOC following infection with a different variant. In the same way, there are cases of clusters of Omicron VOC infections in individuals who received a complete first vaccination program followed by an additional dose of mRNA vaccines, and those who were fully vaccinated who received two doses of COVID-19 (vaccine product not known).

Seroprevalence of the population

Studies conducted on seroepidemiology in the EU/EEA over the past few months have revealed an increase in seropositivity in the population, and Finland having estimates of more than 90%. Finland also has the highest levels of seropositivity are usually from studies carried out among older cohorts that were the first vaccine-free. The majority of studies do not distinguish between vaccine-induced or natural immunity. However, seropositivity statistics closely track patterns in the coverage of vaccines across various cohorts. The increasing rate of seropositivity has been due to vaccination. Knowing the extent of acquired immunity naturally in the general population is challenging without study-based studies. Estimates based on the reported prevalence are susceptible to being inaccurate.

It is possible that the Omicron VOC, and possible future variants that carry multiple mutations, can dramatically reduce or even evade the naturally-induced or vaccine-induced immunity. Therefore, it is essential to have a thorough knowledge of the percentage of people who have natural immunity and immunity to vaccines to evaluate the health risks of variations, such as those of the Omicron VOC. Different serological tests can be used to discern between natural and caused immunity. There have been several studies conducted throughout the European region which have employed these tests; one survey in Geneva that was conducted between the 1st of June 2021 and 7 July 2021 found overall seropositivity of 66.1 percent (64.1-68.0) as well as an infection-induced seroprevalence rate of 29.9 percent. Recent data from a study that tracked blood donors from the UK identified seropositivity rates of 22.7 percent (95 percent CI 95%)

22.0 percent to 23.5 22.0% to 23.5) for the induced antibodies caused by infection, and 97.8 percent for antibodies caused by vaccines or natural infection from 4 October through 29 November 2021.

Prognoses for Omicron VOC Epidemiology

ECDC has created simulations of the anticipated number of deaths for the Omicron VOC compared to Delta VOC for different scenarios from 1 December 2021 to the 31st March 2022. These scenarios reflect the broad spectrum of uncertainty that we currently know about this VOC. The exact date when the Omicron VOC will become dominant will depend on the increase in growth against Delta VOC. Delta VOC, which will differ between the EU/EEA nations. Suppose there are no further steps implemented now. In that case, Omicron will probably become an important strain within the EU/EEA region in February 2022 at the end of the year. It may be in certain particular EU/EEA nations by the end of December 2021 (Figure 6). The figures of Figure 6 could be subject to uncertainty about Omicron's transmissibility as well as its immunity escape, and other variables which are represented as median estimates (black line) and 50% reliable interval (a dark grey area) and 90% reliable interval (a light grey area).

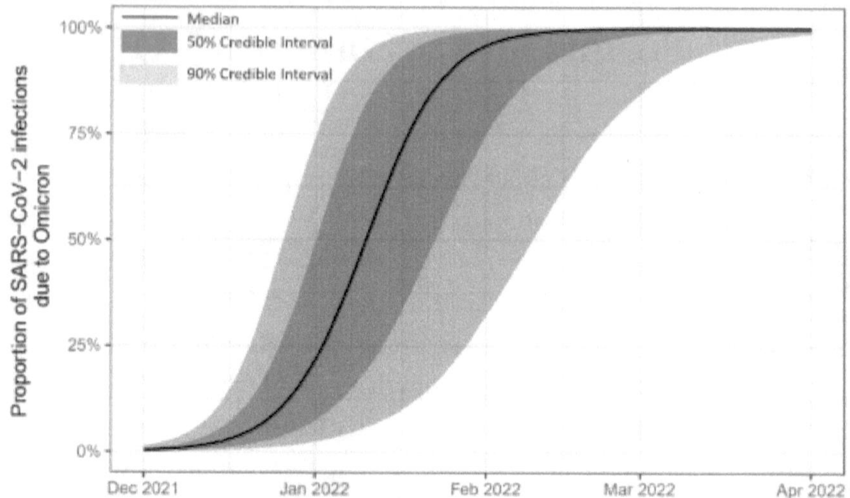

Figure 6. The predicted proportion of SARS-CoV-2-related infections caused by Omicron VOC

Note: The results are based on 50 000 randomly selected samples from the distributions of the benefits of growth for Omicron VOC over the Delta VOC (with the majority of in the range that are -0.2; +0.5); the proportional reduction ineffectiveness of the vaccine due to the escape of immune cells (0.3; 0.6); the proportional decrease of natural immunity (0.5; 0.8); and the proportion that will be Omicron VOC infected individuals on 1 December 2021 (0.1 percent 1.1 percent). We also took values from various levels of vaccination and the natural levels of immunity comparable to the median across EU/EEA countries, having coverage from a range of 40-50 percent and innate immunity between 30 to 60 percent. The level of protection for the population was determined from the measured country-specific values and then averaged across the EU/EEA countries.

Based on the projected future direction predicted for Omicron's future trajectory Omicron VOC, we can expect a decline in the protection offered to all people because of this particular variant. Figure 7 shows the predicted effect of the expanding distribution of Omicron and declining immunity on the average population vaccine effect. The drastic reduction in the vaccine effectiveness could, to a certain degree, be mitigated through mass-scale, high-volume booster vaccination programs. The results shown in figure 7 appear to be following the previous ECDC Rapid risk assessments and threat assessment briefs that strongly recommended booster vaccinations. The need to administer booster doses has significantly increased due to the rapid rise from the Omicron VOC in the EU/EEA.

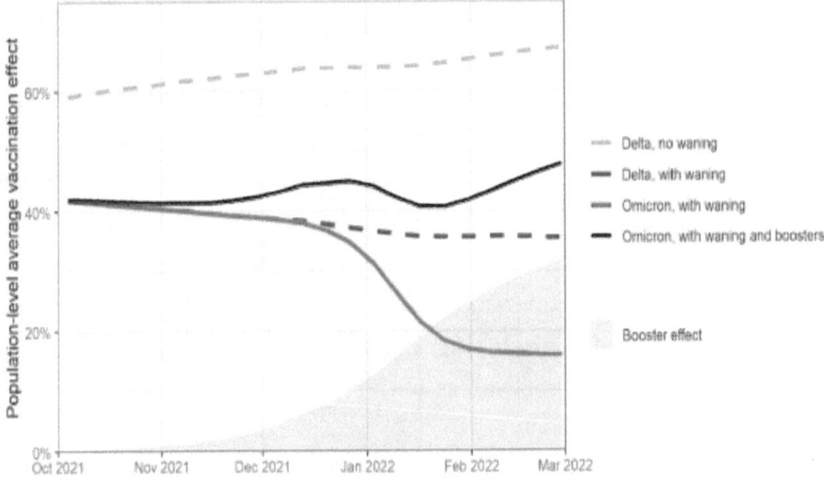

Figure 7. The population-level vaccine effect on infection prevention over time is averaged across all the people in the EU/EEA.

The estimated effect of vaccination on the population level to protect against infections is the mean effect of immunization on the probability of getting ill for the entire population. An amount of 100% means complete protection for all of the people. The grey-dash curve indicates the effect of vaccination (without boosters) in the hypothetical scenario, which ignores the appearance of Omicron and its waning. The red curve that is dashed shows the effect of vaccination (without booster doses) for the hypothetical scenario that involves diminishing the effect, however, without the appearance of Omicron. A solid, red-colored curve illustrates the expected impact of Omicron and the gradual fading of the effects of vaccination (without booster doses for vaccines). The black solid curve depicts similar scenarios to the expected third scenario; however, it also assumes that there is a booster roll-out in those older than 40. In the case of boosters, the rate (boosters daily) that is 60% distribution for second doses is depicted, and the final coverage of booster shots is believed to cover 80% double dose coverage.

In contrast, the effectiveness of vaccines against infection of boosters was estimated to be 90 percent. The shaded area shows the expected effect of boosters, which is equal to the variance of the anticipated Omicron scenario with a fast expansion of boosters (black curve) compared to the anticipated Omicron scenario with no boosters (red curve). The purpose of these graphs is to display approximate trajectories of the order of magnitude, given the large uncertainties in Omicron VOC's spread parameters, the human behavior and country-specific parameters stochasticity, and the simplification of the assumptions used in modelling. In addition, for visualization, the graph shows only the median values with no credible interval within every curve.

In the final analysis, we compared the uncertainties in the Omicron VOC against possible mitigation strategies. We focus on speeding up current COVID-19 vaccine booster programs and reintroducing more stringent non-pharmaceutical interventions to decrease Rt within the EU/EEA region between December 2021 and March 2022. Comparatively to the current state of constant Delta VOC dominance, our findings show that, if the growth benefit of Omicron VOC is not great, an earlier roll-out of boosters can reduce death rates (as is expected). However, if there were no reductions in social contacts, the increase in deaths would be much higher than an initial scenario that reflects the current conditions characterized by Delta VOC dominance (See Figure 8 - Less optimistic scenario). The combination of ongoing booster programs and a greater reduction in social contacts than those already in place in November 2021 may end the increase in deaths. But in higher levels of the assumed Omicron growth benefit that booster programs will not be able to create immunity in the timeframe between December 2021 until March 2022 (Figure 8: Pessimistic, a scenario).

Figure 8. Change in the number of COVID-19-related deaths caused by the dominating Omicron VOC in the EU/EEA between December 2021 and March 2022, when applying a quicker vaccination schedule across various non-pharmaceutical treatments

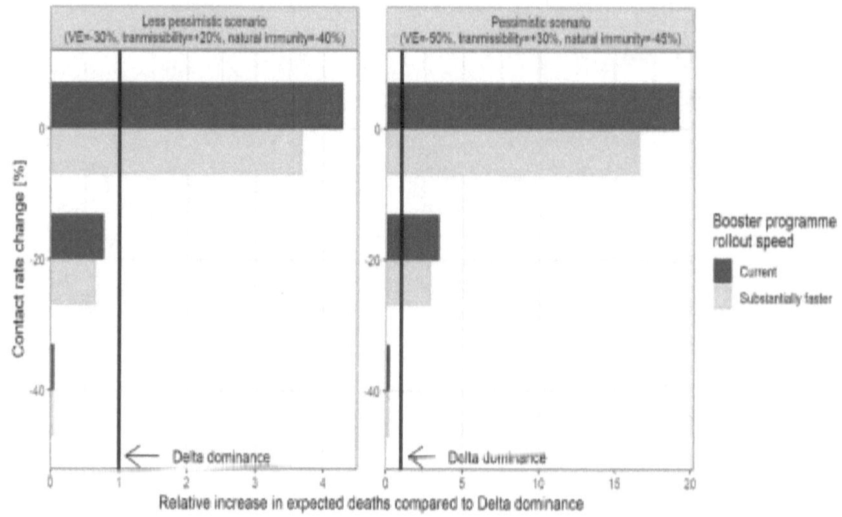

To understand the reinforcement and reintroduction into NPIs that have already been implemented, we assumed that the that Rt was the same as

1.0. Greater transmissibility, lower efficacy (VE) in the case of infection, and less protection for natural immunity because Omicron increases the rate of transmission significantly. The roll-out of vaccinations reflected observed rates across EU/EEA nations, including all booster shots. Since the severity changes are linear, a decrease in Omicron severity could result in a proportional reduction in the excessive seriousness of Omicron as shown in the illustration (e.g., 50 percent decrease in Omicron severity as compared to Delta results in a 50% decrease in the length of the bars over one value and a relative rise in the expected death rate due to Omicron above Delta). Notice that the x-axes of the two figures are different in scale.

The reduction in contact rate could be accomplished through more stringent NPIs.

The results mentioned above from modelling give several clues:

The high rates of SARS-CoV-2 transmission observed at the end of November in 2021 are likely to result in an inevitable increase in burden because of the Delta VOC in many EU/EEA countries through December 2021.

Omicron VOC is likely to be the predominant variant as early as January 2022, but this will depend on the growing advantage and immunity elimination that comes with Omicron VOC.

The level of protection that can be expected at the population level decreases as time passes due to (a) the decline in the immune system induced by vaccines as well as (b) the diminution in the effectiveness of vaccines due to an Omicron VOC (particularly in those individuals who did not receive an Omicron booster).

The Omicron VOC is likely to bring about additional deaths and those predicted by forecasts that only consider the Delta VOC. But, the fatalities will be noticed only at a later time after the Omicron

VOC has taken over (given the delay of some weeks in observing COVID-19 related deaths following SARS-CoV-2 infection diagnosis and generally hospitalization).

The greater the benefit to growth that the Omicron VOC has and its immunity escape and immune escape, the greater the expected burden.

With the Omicron VOC likely being more growth-oriented significant and immediate reductions in the contact rate is required to make sure the COVID-19-related burden remains to a minimum. This is especially relevant given the coming holiday season, which typically involves intergenerational interactions between various households and the potential for super-spreading of events.

The speed of booster vaccination programs is essential to reduce the risk of a burden that could be avoided in early 2022.

The result of staying on the current course and not accelerating (booster) vaccination programs or restriction on contact to lower transmission (bring Rt lower than 1.0) will be the risk of extreme transmission events that could be overwhelming healthcare systems. Also, likely, deaths will not be discovered until 2022, after some time.

Classification of Omicron (B.1.1.529): SARS-CoV-2 Variant of Concern

The Technical Advisory Group on SARS-CoV-2 virus Evolution (TAG-VE) is an expert group that regularly evaluates and monitors the progress of SARS-CoV-2 and evaluates whether specific mutations and combinations alter the behavior in the viral. The TAG-VE met on the 26th of November, 2021, to evaluate the SARS-CoV-2 variant: B.1.1.529.

It is believed that the B.1.1.529 variant was first disclosed by WHO by a patient in South Africa on 24 November 2021. The current epidemiological situation of South Africa has been characterized by three distinct peak levels in cases reported, and the most recent was primarily related to the Delta variant. Recently, infections have been rising rapidly and coincided with the discovery of a B.1.1.529 variant. The first confirmed case of B.1.1.529 condition was detected on the 9th of November 2021.

This variant is characterized by many mutations, a few of which pose a risk. The preliminary evidence suggests a higher risk of re-infections with this variant when opposed to other VOCs. This variant's number of cases is believed to be growing in almost every province in South Africa. Current SARS-CoV-2 diagnostic PCR tests continue to find this variant. Several labs have confirmed that in one commonly used PCR test, there is a possibility that at least one target gene cannot be identified (called S gene dropout or S gene target failure) and can be considered an indicator for this variant subject to confirmation by sequencing. This variant was identified more quickly than other infection outbreaks, suggesting that this variant might possess a potential advantage in growth.

There are many studies in progress, and the TAG-VE continues to study this variation. WHO will share its findings with the Member States and the public when it is required.

Based on evidence that suggests a negative change in the epidemiology of COVID-19, The TAG-VE has advised WHO the variant needs to be identified as a VOC; in addition, the WHO has declared B.1.1.529 as a VOC that is named Omicron.

In this regard, nations are required to perform these things:

- improve surveillance and sequencing efforts to understand the circulating SARS-CoV-2 variants better.
- Submit complete genome sequences and the associated metadata to a public database, like GISAID.
- Report initial clusters or cases of VOC infections to WHO via the IHR method.
- In the event of capacity and collaboration together with other international groups, conduct lab tests and field investigations to better understand the possible impacts of VOC on the COVID-19 epidemic and severity, as well as the effectiveness of social and public health measures, diagnostic techniques, and immune responses, antigen neutralization, and other pertinent features.

The public is reminded of taking steps to decrease the risk of contracting COVID-19, such as known public health and social methods like wearing well-fitting masks and hand hygiene, physical separation, improving the air quality of indoor spaces, and avoiding areas that are crowded, and having a vaccination.

For further reference, **WHO has** working definitions **for SARS-CoV-2 Variant Intent (VOI) and Variant of Concern (VOC).**

A SARS-CoV-2 VoI is a variant of SARS-CoV-2:

- with genetic modifications which are expected or proven to alter the characteristics of viruses like transmission and disease severity, as well as the ability to escape from infection as well as therapeutic or diagnostic escape, and
- It has been recognized as the cause of significant transmission in communities and multiple clusters of COVID-19 across various countries, with an increase in relative frequency, as well as an increasing number of cases or other evident health effects that could indicate the possibility of a new threat for global public health.

The SARS-CoV-2 **VOC** is a variant of SARS-CoV-2 that has the characteristics of a VoI (see earlier) and, by an assessment of comparability, it has been proven to be linked with any or all of the following symptoms in a manner that is of global significance for public health:

- Increased transmission or a negative change in the COVID-19 epidemiology OR
- An increase in virulence, or a change in the clinical presentation of disease OR
- Lower effectiveness of social and health measures, or diagnostics available or vaccines. Therapeutics, diagnostics, and vaccines

How serious are Omicron-related infections?

As the spread of cases increases and nations plan their responses as they spread, scientists are waiting for crucial information regarding the severity of illness due to the variant of coronavirus.

It's been less than four weeks since it was announced that coronavirus with mutations was discovered within southern Africa. Since then, numerous nations around the globe have reported cases of

Omicron and; this includes the alarming amount of cases from people who had either had vaccinations or prior SARS-CoV-2 infection.

However, as politicians and public health officials attempt to plan a path for coming Omicron increases, they have to do this without an exact answer to a crucial issue: how severe will these Omicron illnesses be?

The data aren't as extensive and a bit sloppy. "There is inevitably a lag between infection and hospitalization," says epidemiologist for infectious diseases Mark Woolhouse at the University of Edinburgh, UK. "In the meantime, policy decisions have to be made, and that's not straightforward."

Hospitalization rate

Initial results offer some possibilities. Recent reports of South Africa have consistently noted the lower number of hospitalizations because of Omicron infections than infections due to the Delta variant, which is the current cause for most SARS-CoV-2-related infections worldwide. On December 14, the South African private health insurer Discovery Health in Johannesburg announced that the risk of hospitalization has been 29% lower in people afflicted with Omicron than those infected with an earlier variant.

It has been suggested that Omicron is more prone to causing milder illness than other variations. But, according to researchers, it's too early to know for sure and crucial details regarding the methodological aspects of the study have not yet been released. These details are vital in interpreting the data regarding the severity of the disease, which may be distorted by factors like hospital capacity, the age, and general health of those

The results of Discovery Health are in keeping with other studies conducted across the United States, says Waasila Jassat, a physician and public health specialist in the National Institute for Communicable Diseases in Johannesburg. "There are many caveats and disclaimers around early severity data," she adds. "But the picture is very consistent."

It may take some time for a consistent picture of the disease to emerge from countries that have fewer Omicron cases. On the 13th of December, Denmark published data that showed that the hospitalization rates for those affected by Omicron appeared to be similar to those of people with different variants. However, this analysis was based on just 3400 incidents with Omicron disease and 37 admissions.

A 16 December report from Imperial College London found no indication of decreased hospitalizations resulting from Omicron infections than Delta in England. However, it was based on comparatively only a handful of instances. In the end, the number of cases isn't enough to make definitive conclusions regarding the severity of the disease caused by Omicron, as per Troels Lillebaek, an infectious disease expert at the University of Copenhagen.

The rapid spread of the disease can be a risk to health systems, even if the chance of a severe illness or death is small for each individual. "A small fraction of a very large number is still a large number," Woolhouse states. Woolhouse. "So, the population-level threat is very real."

South Africa's positive data may not mean that Omicron is less harmful than other variants. Over 70% of people in areas with high levels of Omicron have previously been exposed to SARS-CoV-2, and around 40% of them have had at minimum one dose of COVID-19 vaccine, according to Jassat. This makes it challenging to discern the effects of pre-existing immunity from the inherent characteristics of the virus itself.

Vaccine protection

Research has revealed that Omicron could be able to bypass certain COVID immune system-distributed vaccines, as well as early findings obtained from the UK Health Security Agency suggest that the vaccines may not be as effective in preventing Omicron infections like they were for other types, even though the number of cases examined was insufficient to make a definitive determination of how much protection diminished.

However, vaccinations can keep the majority of recipients from serious illness and death caused by COVID-19. Apart from antibodies to fight infection, the previously infected or vaccinated immune system creates T cells that recognize viruses and eliminate virus-infected cells, possibly limiting the extent of the infection.

Researchers have traced Omicron's panoply of mutations into the SARS-CoV-2 protein fragments recognized by T cells after natural infection and vaccination. They discovered no mutations in the majority of the fragments. When it comes to immunization, over 70 percent of the fragments remain 100% intact, according to Immunologist Alessandro Sette at the La Jolla Institute for Immunology in California.

There's still work to be done; scientists are already carrying out tests in the lab to see how T cells that are generated in response to vaccinations and infection with different varieties react with Omicron. The results are expected within the next few weeks. "I'm optimistic that the reactivity is going to be preserved, at least in part," Sette states. "How much of it will be preserved remains to be seen."

There isn't a method to draw a clear line connecting the level of T-cell reactivity and the protection against severe illness. Recent studies have revealed that T-cell responses to SARS-CoV-2 have been linked to less viral load and less severe disease, but they do not define a threshold at the point that this protection could start to diminish,

Sette says. It will ultimately boil down to waiting for information on deaths and hospitalizations from Omicron.

Children are at risk of contracting infections

As these results are released, the researchers will look specifically at the effects of Omicron in children. Findings from South Africa have suggested that hospitalization rates for children afflicted with Omicron are much higher than those observed in previous waves. However, researchers warn that this does not indicate that the children will be more susceptible to Omicron as they were exposed to Delta and other variations. Jassat states that children have lower coronavirus infections and vaccines than adulthood, which means their levels of prior immunity aren't as strong.

Hospitalization rates higher in children in the initial phases of an outbreak might be a sign of increased capacity at the hospital, allowing a child to stay in the hospital for observation, who would otherwise be removed from the hospital, she states.

The environment in which children are exposed could play a role in this: prolonged exposures at home with an infected parent can result in an increased risk of contracting the disease than a brief exposure at school, claims David Dowdy, an infectious-disease epidemiologist at the Johns Hopkins Bloomberg School of Public Health in Baltimore, Maryland. "Everyone is focused on the pathogen here," the doctor declares. "But it's not just about the variant, and it's also about the host and the environment."

Risk communication

Omicron VOC vs Delta VOC

While much attention is paid to Omicron VOC, it is important to remember that while there are many concerns, it is essential to remind everyone that the primary danger is Delta. Although there is a lot of uncertainty in the scientific literature regarding the various aspects of Omicron but the potentially devastating negative impact of Delta is well-known. Therefore, information must be disseminated widely to encourage vaccinations and appropriate non-pharmaceutical treatments. This is particularly important during the lead-up to the holiday season, as the increased festivities and travel can make conditions conducive to a high level of infection. Also, it is important to be reminded that an increase in COVID-19 hospitalizations doesn't just pose a serious challenge to health care systems but can also negatively impact the treatment and care for other illnesses.

In the long run, it is important to focus on enhancing people's motivation to stick to protection rules for a long time (both the vaccination process and non-prescription drugs). There is a good chance that certain measures are required for a few months in the future. The risk communication strategies must consider the variety of possible social, economic, and political impacts that they might have on society.

The message about vaccination

Regarding the lack of evidence regarding the Omicron variant and the uncertainty concerning the immune escape issue about the COVID-19 vaccines currently available (and treatments), it is imperative to communicate the importance of remaining completely vaccinated looking for an extra or booster dose is essential. It is essential to constantly communicate about the safety and efficacy of COVID-19 vaccinations and emphasize the vital role that COVID-19 vaccines have played in preventing serious illness, hospitalization, and even deaths since the beginning of vaccination campaigns. To do this, it's important to share the findings of research studies that have examined the efficacy and effectiveness of COVID-19 vaccination programs. In the earlier part of the document, this is the evidence of how deaths and hospitalizations are greatly reduced in countries with high levels of vaccination and the evidence that people who are fully vaccinated and suffer from breakthrough illnesses are at significantly less chance of contracting a severe disease or requiring hospitalization than people who have not been vaccinated. Visualization of data is an effective method to convey these messages. The public needs to be assured about the effectiveness and power of the COVID-19 vaccines currently available even if adjustments to vaccination strategies are necessary (e.g., the administration of a booster dose or another dose of COVID-19) and despite the necessity of maintaining the NPIs at a certain amount due to the significant number of COVID-19 patients.

Additionally, the general public might have questions and doubts about the necessity of vaccines in the face of the flood of information about the potential impact on this Omicron VOC, especially when there is an over-interpretation or selective interpretation of the results of recent studies. It is essential to understand this because scientific research is a process that takes time. Further studies and evidence from real life will be required before definitive conclusions can be drawn.

There is always new evidence, so messages about possible revisions to vaccines or the necessity for further boosters should be clear about the current uncertainty to prevent future confusion.

Recognizing and correcting misinformation

Like it has happened many times throughout the COVID-19 outbreak, where there was scientific uncertainty or gaps in information, and the rise of Omicron could spread false information. In the countries where online social listening is not commonly practiced (to detect rumours that circulate and misperceptions, which can later be dealt with via risk communication), National authorities might be interested in investing in this crucial field.

The reporting of data to ECDC

It is vital to evaluate the effectiveness of COVID-19 vaccinations with future study designs, in which adjustments are possible for the majority of confounding factors; it is also possible to evaluate the effectiveness of vaccines in outbreak situations. The data from these rapid studies may be of particular importance in light of the latest questions regarding the efficacy of vaccines (e.g., studies involving the development of VOCs). Studies involving emerging VOCs can be collected quickly and provide preliminary or additional evidence to support other estimates. The advantage of conducting outbreak studies is that in certain settings (e.g., schools), vaccine records could be easily accessible. The investigation can be conducted in conjunction with implementing measures to control.

With this aim, ECDC has published and advocates using a generic protocol that is intended to be adapted to local/national contexts to guide the implementation of vaccine effectiveness studies against SARS-CoV-2 infection (on the occurrence of an outbreak in semi-closed-settings). Two studies and their methods are proposed as cohort studies and case-control studies. Semi-closed environments are situations where the enrolment/employment lists can easily identify the inhabitants (e.g., schools, other educational institutions, or workplaces). ECDC is considering the possibility of reporting voluntary outbreak-related information within EpiPulse as described by this report and providing an efficient initial analysis of the effect estimates in connection with the emergence of CoV-2 SARS variant Omicron.

Measures to travel

Evidence shows that the Omicron VOC has already been introduced to several EU/EEA countries, and some are already experiencing transmission through the community. Travel restrictions for the first days of the detection and recognition that the VOC was Omicron have been designed to give the public time to the hope of better understanding its specific characteristics and deal with the high current flow of the Delta VOC across EU/EEA countries. Measures to prevent travel (e.g., travel restrictions or other measures) must be evaluated according to the current epidemiological situation and the recommendations in the "Testing" section above.

To avoid transmission of SARS-CoV-2 when traveling, precautions include advising against travel with COVID-19 symptoms and maintenance of NPI measures at transportation hubs and while traveling e.g.

To reduce crowding, paying attention to physical distancing, wearing masks for face protection during travel, adequate ventilation, and so on.) and using recognized EU digital COVID-19 certificates to avoid crowds, keeping a close eye on the road, and using COVID.

For countries who are experiencing their first import Omicron cases and are trying to deter any further introductions of the Omicron VOC from regions with an extremely high rate of community transmission In addition to the advice above and pre-departure tests (preferably an RT-PCR test for at least 48 hours before travel or RADT at least 24 hours before departure) or tests and quarantine after arrival can be considered by travellers who come from regions with the highest level of community-based transmission Omicron VOC. With the evidence that the Omicron VOC has been introduced into various EU/EEA countries and some countries already experiencing community transmission, the aforementioned measures will likely not be needed for long.

It is essential to ensure that the public has access to information about the current situation. Health precautions are available to travellers to increase awareness and encourage compliance. Furthermore, healthcare professionals' understanding is crucial to ensure that any suspect cases of COVID-19 that present to health establishments have a complete medical record taken. Suppose any cases are discovered among travellers from areas prone to transmission by the community or where the epidemiological condition is unclear; the isolation process and contact tracer testing should be performed with care (see the section above). The virus isolates from these cases must be screened before sequencing to identify the instances of the newly discovered variant.

New variants discovered in EU/EEA countries must be reported every week through the European Surveillance System (TESSy). TESSy permits reporting of cases that involve the VOC Omicron or cases with the deletion of the S-gene both via variant-data or case-based data.